Kathleen Kendall-Tackett, PhD, IBCLC

Depression
in New Mothers
Causes, Consequences,
and Treatment Alternatives

*Pre-publication
REVIEWS,
COMMENTARIES,
EVALUATIONS . . .*

"*Depression in New Mothers: Causes Consequences and Treatment Alternatives* by Kathleen Kendall-Tackett carefully describes the complex landscape of postpartum depression. Her evidence-based, cogent examination of the life threads, biological possibilities, and realities of new motherhood encourage the reader to abandon simplistic or one-dimensional explanations for this common and potentially devastating life event.

Without a doubt, this book is a must-read for anyone working with childbearing women. The mothers we serve deserve nothing less than knowledgeable, prepared practitioners."

Karin Cadwell, PhD, RN, IBCLC
*Faculty, Healthy Children Project,
East Sandwich, Massachusetts;
Adjunct Faculty, The Union Institute
& University, Cincinnati, Ohio*

"Depression in new mothers is a tip-of-the-iceberg issue with profound implications for the woman (of course), her baby, other children, and the entire family. Dr. Kathleen Kendall-Tackett reminds us that 'becoming a mother turns a woman's world upside down.'

Something is very wrong with our care and support of women if almost 20 percent of new mothers are clinically depressed, suffer postpartum anxiety and obsessive-compulsive disorders, and/or endure post-traumatic stress disorders after giving birth. Even though these reactions to bearing a child may be commonplace, they are not normal. Effective treatments are available that support breastfeeding and the mother-baby relationship. This stunning compendium of research evidence, clinical descriptions, and real-life stories is a must-have resource for all professionals working in the field of maternal and child health."

Linda J. Smith, BSE, IBCLC
*Director, Bright Future Lactation
Resource Centre Ltd.
Dayton, Ohio*

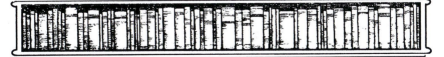

Depression in New Mothers
Causes, Consequences, and Treatment Alternatives

Depression
in New Mothers
Causes, Consequences,
and Treatment Alternatives

Kathleen Kendall-Tackett, PhD, IBCLC

The Haworth Maltreatment and Trauma Press®
An Imprint of The Haworth Press, Inc.
New York • London • Oxford

For more information on this book or to order, visit
http://www.haworthpress.com/store/product.asp?sku=5230

or call 1-800-HAWORTH (800-429-6784) in the United States and Canada
or (607) 722-5857 outside the United States and Canada

or contact orders@HaworthPress.com

Published by

The Haworth Maltreatment and Trauma Press®, an imprint of The Haworth Press, Inc., 10 Alice Street, Binghamton, NY 13904-1580.

PUBLISHER'S NOTE
Identities and circumstances of individuals discussed in this book have been changed to protect confidentiality.

Cover design by Marylouise E. Doyle.

Library of Congress Cataloging-in-Publication Data

Kendall-Tackett, Kathleen A.
    Depression in new mothers : causes, consequences, and treatment alternatives / Kathleen Kendall-Tackett.
        p. ; cm.
    Includes bibliographical references and index.
    ISBN-13: 978-0-7890-1838-0 (hard : alk. paper)
    ISBN-10: 0-7890-1838-1 (hard : alk. paper)
    ISBN-13: 978-0-7890-1839-7 (soft : alk. paper)
    ISBN-10: 0-7890-1839-X (soft : alk. paper)
    1. Postpartum depression. 2. Postpartum depression—Risk factors. 3. Postpartum depression—Treatment.
    [DNLM: 1. Depression, Postpartum—diagnosis. 2. Depression, Postpartum—etiology. 3. Depression, Postpartum—therapy. 4. Maternal Welfare—psychology. 5. Risk Factors. 6. Socioeconomic Factors. WQ 500 K33d 2005] I. Title.
    RG852.K448 2005
    618.7'6—dc22
                                                                                            2004022688

CONTENTS

ABOUT THE AUTHOR

Kathleen Kendall-Tackett, PhD, IBCLC, is a health psychologist, an International Board Certified Lactation Consultant, a Research Associate Professor at the University of New Hampshire's Family Research Lab, and a Fellow of the American Psychological Association. She is widely published in the fields of family violence, maternal depression, perinatal health, and disability. Dr. Kendall-Tackett is a La Leche League leader and serves as La Leche League Professional Liaison for Maine and New Hampshire. She is also Chair of the New Hampshire Breastfeeding Taskforce. Dr. Kendall-Tackett is the author or editor of ten books, including *The Hidden Feelings of Motherhood, The Well-Ordered Home, Treating the Lifetime Health Effects of Childhood Victimization,* and *The Health Consequences of Abuse in the Family.* She has won several awards, including the Outstanding Research Study Award from the American Professional Society on the Abuse of Children, and most recently was named 2003 Distinguished Alumna by the College of Behavioral and Social Sciences, California State University, Chico. She lives in New Hampshire with her husband Doug Tackett, her sons Ken and Chris, and quite a few pets.

Foreword

> To be conscious that you are ignorant is a great step
> to knowledge.
>
> Benjamin Disraeli

Denial and ignorance are two of the barriers in recognizing and treating women suffering from perinatal mood disorders. After a quarter century in the field, I see much less public denial surrounding this topic but, sadly, people remain appallingly ignorant. I believe that knowledge is power. Without accurate information we become passive victims. To become more knowledgeable, we need more books describing up-to-date, research-based studies. *Depression in New Mothers: Causes, Consequences, and Treatment Alternatives* provides us with more than statistics and information. This is book has a heart. It is written by a mother who understands motherhood. The reader's knowledge quotient is going to increase dramatically from reading this landmark contribution to the literature.

Kathleen Kendall-Tackett has been a pioneer educator in the field of maternal mental health since her first book, *Postpartum Depression,* was published in 1993. In this new volume, she expands upon her knowledge of the complexities and interrelationships in the field of maternal depression. Her goal is to equip her readers with the information needed to make a real difference in the lives of mothers and babies. She has achieved this goal through a systematic framework that will help readers understand the topic and how to communicate effectively with postpartum mothers.

Myths about motherhood are also barriers to seeking appropriate care during pregnancy and the postpartum period. The author has identified four distinct pervasive myths about postpartum depression. Misperceptions about depression are dangerous! We cannot effectively provide adequate assistance if health care providers and the public continue to perpetuate them. In Chapter 2, she demonstrates how expensive myths are because of the harm untreated depression causes to mother and baby. We cannot afford not to get involved. I agree with her message that we must get serious, seek the truth, and act on this knowledge.

Each chapter in *Depression in New Mothers* has summaries of thought-provoking international research studies. The depth of the science is staggering and fascinating. We still do not understand all that neuroscience tells us about the brain, but we have many clues. When I was first exposed to postpartum psychiatric illness in 1984 it was described as a "picture puzzle." The pieces are beginning to fit together and at the same time we continue to ask more questions. For example, what comes first, depression or fatigue? Kendall-Tackett tackles those issues by presenting the underpinnings of fatigue, the immune system, cholesterol levels, and pain. She asks excellent questions about the role of breastfeeding cessation and depression. Which comes first? In Chapter 4, the issues of negative birth experience and untreated previous trauma are given the attention they deserve. Women need time and a safe, trusting environment to share their nightmares. If we dare to inquire, what will we do with this information? Maybe we will save lives and relationships. As the author reminds us, recovery from trauma is achievable.

The topic of infant characteristics and depression in their mothers as described in Chapter 5 is not discussed often enough. Infant crying, sleep habits, prematurity, chronic illness, or disability can also affect mothers' moods. This seems rather obvious, but for years developmental psychologists dismissed their importance. Another reason for this "disconnect" was because the researchers and clinicians in reproductive and infant psychology were not sharing their findings with the scientists actively researching postpartum psychiatric illness and vice versa. Fortunately, this has changed. If your professional interest is the baby, my hope is that you will begin to turn your attention to the mother's emotional needs as well. The baby needs her to be healthy. Make certain that she is not still grieving for the baby she perceived would be born without special challenges. Look into her eyes with an open heart, and ask a caring question about how she is feeling.

Chapters 6 and 7 delve into the psychological and social components of postpartum depression. The author summarizes the large body of literature on the psychological factors involved, including self-esteem, self-efficacy, and expectations. In addition, she describes research on previous psychiatric history, depression during pregnancy, violence against women, the connection between childhood and domestic abuse, parenting difficulties, abuse and breastfeeding, and loss. Since my personal bias is toward social risk factors, I could not agree more with her sentence "women do not become mothers in a vacuum." She offers an insightful summary of all the known risk factors in Table 7.1. Her concept asks what supports or hinders the mother-infant relationship. We do know what hurts and what helps. This leads to the book's final chapters on assessment and treatment.

A major challenge facing us is a mother's own denial. I have spoken on the telephone with depressed mothers for more than twenty-five years. These women are not in denial and, frankly, I do not worry about them. I am deeply troubled, however, with our inability to engage in a dialogue with those who never reach out for help. Plainly put, we cannot treat her if she does not perceive any need. And I speak from personal experience as well. My own denial lasted far too long. It is very tricky. But again, I believe that education is the key. If we can routinely start talking about negative emotions related to childbearing as naturally as we do pain in labor and sore nipples, then there will be progress in improving maternal mental health.

Chapters 9, 10, and 11 offer comprehensive descriptions of alternative and complementary medical treatments, including psychotherapy, community interventions and psychoactive substances. Kendall-Tackett covers each of these thoroughly, citing the most recent research. Mothers ask me, "What can I take?" "Do I have to take medicine?" Some state emphatically, "I won't take anything." I do not have a medical background, and yet by having a better understanding of antidepressants, I can direct mothers toward learning about their treatment options. We are beginning to learn what treatments do work, but since the science has not given us answers to fully comprehend what is wrong, our clinical experience is rather hit and miss. Yes, we can make our mothers well, but major gaps in understanding still exist.

After reading so much science, it is both touching and refreshing to conclude with the words of one mother, Jenny, who has "been there." There is no substitute for truth and honesty. When it comes to feeling equipped to help others, it truly begins with being satisfied that you know your own comfort level with mental illness. It is my hope that after reading this important book readers will indeed be ready to make a difference in the lives of mothers and babies. Kathleen Kendall-Tackett, as author and educator, surely is an inspiration to all of us.

Jane Honikman, Founding Director
Postpartum Support International
Santa Barbara, California

Preface

The world has changed since 1991. That was when I sat down to write the first version of this book. I was a new mother with a recently acquired PhD in developmental psychology. In trying to make sense of my own postpartum experience, I started to read the research literature on postpartum depression. I was stunned at how different it was from what I was reading in the popular press. Articles for mothers complained that no one was studying this topic, especially in the United States. Both parts of that statement were demonstrably false. At that time, I found approximately 200 articles, and some of the best research was conducted in the United States.

Popular articles also repeatedly attributed depression to hormonal fluctuations. But empirical support for this theory was surprisingly weak. There was, however, a great deal of support for variables such as social support, infant temperament, and previous episodes of depression. I realized that depression in new mothers was far more complex and far more interesting than I had realized. Armed with this knowledge, I put together a book proposal. The rest, as they say, is history.

Since the publication of *Postpartum Depression* (Sage, 1993), the field has also evolved. When I first started, there was little interest in depression in new mothers. That has changed. Over the past fourteen years, I've conducted training for thousands of health care professionals across the United States. I've continued to learn. At almost every conference, someone had an excellent question that sent me back to the literature to find the answer.

I have also had a lot more contact with mothers than when I wrote the earlier text. My contact with mothers came via my work as a breastfeeding counselor and later as a board-certified lactation consultant. Often my role was to help them sort out their treatment options and find a plan that allowed them to continue to breastfeed their babies. I have also talked with mothers as they dealt with issues of past abuse, overwhelming fatigue, work and family issues, and children with special needs. My contact with mothers led me to write a book specifically for them: *The Hidden Feelings of Motherhood* (Pharmasoft, 2005).

When I first started to work on this book, I was pleased by what I found. Where once I found hundreds of articles, now I found thousands. The study of depression in new mothers has also gained in sophistication and complexity. For example, in the first book, I had to pull from other literatures to be able to talk about the impact of postpartum pain on depression, or the impact of negative birth experiences. Now studies exist specifically on these topics. Another striking feature of the more recent literature is its international scope. Studies come from literally around the world. The Internet has, of course, made access to these articles easier than ever. In addition, the studies of assessment and treatment are recent—and welcome—additions to this literature.

The book you are about to read is essentially a new text. I have preserved some of the studies cited in the original for continuity and because they are good studies. In working on the first book, I also had many opportunities to interview mothers in depth. I have included their stories from the original because they are timeless and continue to illustrate points in a way that no mere review of the literature can.

Conference participants often tell me that the topic of depression in new mothers is more interesting than they imagined. I hope that this will be true for you as well. I also want to encourage to you get involved with this population. No matter what your role, there is a way you can help. The late Ray Helfer once described the perinatal period as a "window of opportunity" in our work with families. You have before you an opportunity to make a real difference in the lives of mothers and babies. My goal is to equip you to do just that.

Acknowledgments

This book is the result of many people's efforts. I'd like to first thank my colleague, friend, and editor Bob Geffner for his help with this project and guiding it through the proposal and publication process. I would also like to thank the many mothers who have shared their stories with me, who have written back to tell me about their recovery, and who continue to amaze me with their generosity of spirit. I would not be in this field without them.

Researchers from around the world were kind enough to share their latest research with me, answering my questions, e-mailing me articles, and simply providing a fantastic wealth of information for me to mine. My heartfelt thanks to Cheryl Beck, Marjorie Beeghley, Jane Fisher, Joan Webster, Peter Cooper, Michael O'Hara, Deb Issokson, Mary Benedict, Ed Tronick, Katherine Weinberg, and the many others who have contributed to the knowledge base on perinatal health.

I would also like to thank Jane Honikman and Larry Kruckman of Postpartum Support International, who helped lead me to mothers. As always, I am also grateful to many individual La Leche League leaders and the organization they represent: La Leche League International. They continue to make a difference for mothers around the world. I am proud to be a part of it.

I received valuable advice on my chapters on treatments for depression from the following individuals: Thomas Hale, PhD; Tieraona Low Dog, MD; Nina Iselin, ND; and Melissa Bernadin. I thank all of them for their timely input and suggestions.

I would also like to thank my co-laborers at the Family Research Laboratory, including Sarah Giacomoni, Kelly Foster, Doreen Cole, and Vicki Benn. I especially thank them for their careful work on behalf of children and families, the great questions they ask, and for making me laugh.

As always, I thank my family as we slogged through another book together. My husband, Doug, and sons, Ken and Chris, are the joys of my life. I thank them for always being there, encouraging me to take periodic breaks, and teaching me about what a family can be. I love them all.

The mother is the most precious possession of the nation, so precious that society advances its highest well-being when it protects the functions of the mother.

Ellen Key (1846-1926)

Chapter 1

Depression in New Mothers: Myths versus Reality

We have all seen the pictures. The attractive young woman holding her angelic sleeping baby. Her house is spotless; her handsome and adoring husband is nearby. As attractive as this image is, it is far from the reality that many new mothers face. Some women find their transition to motherhood less than smooth. They may feel overwhelmed, isolated, and depressed (Beck, 2002).

Postpartum depression isolates mothers when they most need the help of others. Mothers may be ashamed to admit that life with a new baby is not always bliss. They may assume that everyone has made a smoother transition to motherhood than they have. They may be truly embarrassed that they are not able to cope better.

MYTHS ABOUT POSTPARTUM DEPRESSION

Unfortunately, people have many misperceptions about depression in new mothers. These myths can keep mothers from receiving the attention they need. Here are some of the most common.

Myth #1: Depression in New Mothers Is Not Serious

One of the most prevalent myths is that postpartum depression is not serious. Fewer people voice this myth today in the wake of the Andrea Yates case. Andrea Yates was the mother in Texas who drowned her five young children in the bathtub while suffering from both postpartum depression and psychosis. She was convicted of murder. I describe her story in more detail in Chapter 2.

Many fail to realize that depression that does not end in infanticide can still be harmful to both mothers and babies. I visit this topic again in Chapter 2.

Myth #2: Postpartum Depression Is More Common in White Middle-Class Women

There is a prevailing belief that postpartum depression is something that only afflicts affluent white women (Martinez, Johnston-Robledo, Ulsh, & Chrisler, 2000).

Revelations of postpartum depression by such well-known women as Princess Diana and Marie Osmond, although helpful in one sense, have reinforced the notion that postpartum depression is a condition of privilege. Yet, as you shall see, postpartum depression affects women in many different cultures and at all income levels.

Myth #3: Postpartum Depression Will Go Away on Its Own

Unfortunately, untreated postpartum depression can last for months or even longer. Zelkowitz and Milet (2001) identified forty-eight couples in which one or both partners was suffering from postpartum mental illness. Four months later, 54 percent of the mothers and 60 percent of their partners still had psychiatric diagnoses. In a second study, mothers were assessed at two, three, six, and twelve months postpartum. Mothers depressed at two months continued to be depressed at each subsequent assessment point throughout the first year (Beeghly et al., 2002).

Myth #4: Women with Postpartum Depression Cannot Breastfeed

Sadly, many women, when they seek help for depression, are told that they must wean their babies so they can take medications. For some mothers, weaning is no problem. But for others, abrupt weaning is experienced as a significant loss. The good news is that many treatments are compatible with breastfeeding. They are described in Chapters 9 to 11.

ASSUMPTIONS ABOUT POSTPARTUM DEPRESSION

So how do we begin to think about postpartum depression? I have developed a framework that has been helpful in my work with new mothers. It provides a way of talking with mothers about what is going on in their lives and for understanding their responses.

Becoming a Mother Is a Stressful Life Event

This first assumption seems obvious in one way, but we often do not keep it in mind. We need to acknowledge that becoming a mother turns a woman's world upside down. It changes almost every aspect of her life: her work, her home, and even her ability to do something as simple as taking a shower. This is not to say that it is a negative event. But we must acknowledge that the transition to motherhood can cause a great deal of stress.

Depression Is Within the Normal Range of Responses Following a Stressful Event

We also need to acknowledge that when exposed to a stressful life event, a certain percentage of people are going to become depressed. This assumption is helpful because it normalizes depression. (But that is different than saying it is of no consequence.) When we accept that depression can be part of life, it makes it more comfortable for us to discuss with mothers. On the other hand, if we treat depression as a freak occurrence, we are going to be uncomfortable, and the mother is likely to feel shame.

The Causes of Postpartum Depression Vary from Woman to Woman

It is also important to keep in mind that postpartum depression has many possible causes. There is no one-size-fits-all explanation for depression in new mothers. The factors underlying postpartum depression vary from woman to woman, and understanding the multiple causes allows us to be more targeted with our interventions.

Postpartum Depression Is Not Limited to the First Six Weeks Postpartum but Can Occur Any Time in the First Year

Some people think that "postpartum" only includes the first four to six weeks after birth. But this is not the way it is described in the research literature. "Postpartum" includes the entire first year (Beck, 1993). We should not be surprised that a woman with a four-month-old, or a nine- or ten-month-old, is depressed. For example, mothers of premature or critically ill babies often become depressed once their babies are out of crisis.

SYMPTOMS OF DEPRESSION

Postpartum depression can manifest in a wide variety of symptoms, including moods of sadness, anhedonia (the inability to experience pleasure), low self-esteem, apathy and social withdrawal, excessive emotional sensitivity, pessimistic thinking, irritability, sleep disturbance, appetite disturbance, impaired concentration, and agitation. These symptoms are common to other forms of depression as well (Beck, 1992; Preston & Johnson, 2001; Rapkin, Mikacich, Moatakef-lmani, & Rasgon, 2002).

Mothers themselves have described a mental "fogginess" that influences their ability to concentrate. This fogginess also impacted their motor skills, so that even running an errand became difficult (Beck, 1993, 2002). Mothers also described anxiety, anger, and guilt, and that they were overwhelmed by the responsibilities of new motherhood (Beck, 2002). They also had a pervasive fear that their lives would never be normal again.

When discussing symptoms of depression in a new mother, some are especially concerning:

- She reports that she has not slept in two to three days.
- She is losing weight rapidly.
- She cannot get out of bed.
- She is ignoring basic grooming.
- She seems hopeless.
- She says that her children would be better off without her.

- She is actively abusing substances.
- She makes strange or bizarre statements (e.g., plans to give her children to strangers).

Diagnostic Criteria for Major Depressive Disorder

Although many mothers may exhibit symptoms of depression, major depression is a more serious manifestation of depressive symptoms that has specific diagnostic criteria. For a diagnosis of major depression, patients must have at least five of the following symptoms during the same two-week period.

1. Depressed mood most of the day
2. Anhedonia most of the day
3. Significant weight loss when not dieting, or weight gain, or change in appetite
4. Insomnia or hypersomnia
5. Psychomotor agitation or retardation
6. Fatigue or loss of energy
7. Feelings of worthlessness or excessive guilt
8. Diminished ability to think or concentrate or make decisions
9. Recurrent thoughts of death, or recurrent suicidal ideation, with or without a specific plan (Reprinted with permission from the *Diagnostic and Statistical Manual of Mental Disorders,* Fourth Edition, Text Revision [Copyright 2000]. American Psychiatric Association, p. 356.)

These symptoms must represent a change from previous functioning, and must include at least depressed mood and anhedonia. These symptoms can be recorded by subjective report or observation of others, and must occur nearly every day (American Psychiatric Association, 2000).

Even depression that does not fill diagnostic criteria, however, should not be ignored. In one study, Weinberg and colleagues (2001) compared women with subclinical depression to three groups: depressed pregnant women, women with postpartum major depression, and nondepressed women. Women with subclinical depression had poorer psychosocial functioning than nondepressed women and were comparable to those with major depression. Moreover, they had more negative and less positive affect, poorer self-esteem, and less confidence as mothers. Dawn describes how her symptoms came on suddenly after the birth of her daughter.

I never really went into labor. They did three inductions. . . . I knew I was going to have a c-section. . . . When they said it was a girl, I just went numb. I just didn't feel like I had given birth. I felt disconnected from my body. I was up for twenty-four hours. I was crying hysterically. She wanted to eat a lot. I never was able to breastfeed. I was in the hospital crying. I didn't feel like her mother. I was very disconnected. I was freaking out. My friends kept telling me that it was the baby blues.

Is Postpartum Depression a Distinct Condition?

When discussing postpartum depression, professionals frequently raise the question of whether it is distinct from nonpuerperal mental illness. By and large, the mental health community acts as if it is not. Some have argued that puerperal and nonpuerperal mental illnesses are similar in terms of their symptomatology and factors predicting onset, and that the only distinguishing characteristic of puerperal mental illness is an onset and triggers that are specific to new motherhood (e.g., infant characteristics, sleep deprivation, and birth experience). Furthermore, at present, there is no specific diagnostic category for postpartum illness in the American Psychiatric Association's (2000) *Diagnostic and Statistical Manual of Mental Disorders,* Fourth Edition, Text Revision (DSM-IV-TR). However, the specifier "with postpartum onset" can be added to the following conditions: major depressive disorder, manic or mixed episode in major depressive disorder, bipolar I or II disorder, or brief psychotic disorder if these conditions occur in the first four weeks after birth (Rapkin et al., 2002).

INCIDENCE

Incidence of postpartum depression is typically 10 to 20 percent of new mothers (Cooper & Murray, 1998; Miller, 2002; Rapkin et al., 2002). Some studies, however, give higher percentages depending on the sample, how depression is defined, and when the measures were taken. If the "depressed" group in a study included those with depressive symptoms, then the percentage of mothers is going to be higher than if only women with a formal diagnosis of major depression are included. Similarly, the percentage will be higher if those with major and minor depression are included in the depressed group. For example, in a sample of 150 women at twelve weeks postpartum, Beck and Gable (2001b) found that 12 percent had major depression and another 19 percent had minor depression. Had both been grouped together, 31 percent of the sample would be in the depressed group.

International Incidence of Postpartum Depression

As I described earlier, postpartum depression is not limited to white middle-class American women (O'Hara, 1994). It is relatively common in other countries as well. For example, in a study of mothers from Costa Rica and Chile, one-third of the mothers were dysphoric after childbirth, and 35 to 50 percent had had at least one episode of major depressive disorder (MDD) in their lifetimes. All the mothers were low-income and had at least one child under the age of three (Wolf, De Andraca, & Lozoff, 2002).

In a sample of 892 women from nine countries, the rates of depression were highest in nonwhites from Asia and South America (Affonso, De, Horowitz, & Mayberry, 2000). Europeans and Australians had the lowest rates. The rate for American mothers was somewhere in between. The countries included were the United States, Guyana, Italy, Sweden, Finland, Korea, Taiwan, India, and Australia.

Mothers in Turkey also experienced postpartum depression at a rate comparable to middle-class American samples. In this study, 14 percent of 257 mothers were depressed at six months postpartum. Risk factors for depression included a higher number of living children, living in a shanty, being an immigrant, having a baby with a serious health problem, a previous history of psychiatric illness for the mother or her husband, and poor relationships with her spouse or his family. The relationship with the husband's family may be particularly salient for women in traditional cultures that are often living with them (Danaci, Dinc, Deveci, Sen, & Icelli, 2002).

Mothers in India ($N = 252$) also suffered from postpartum depression. They were interviewed during their third trimester and at six to eight weeks and six months postpartum. Of these women, 23 percent were depressed, and 78 percent had "substantial" clinical morbidity. Their risk factors for depression included economic deprivation, poor marital relationships, and gender of the infant. These risk factors were similar to those of Western samples, especially poverty and poor marital relationships (see Chapter 7). The factor unique to this culture was gender of the infant; mothers were more likely to become depressed if they had a girl (Patel, Rodrigues, & DeSouza, 2002).

Mothers in Nepal had surprisingly low rates of depression (Regmi, Sligl, Carter, Grut, & Seear, 2002): 12 percent at two to three months postpartum. The authors expressed surprise at this low rate and pointed out that Nepal is one of the poorest countries in the world, with an infant mortality rate of 75 per 1,000.

Finally, in a small sample of Vietnamese and Hmong women living in the United States ($N = 30$), 43 percent were clinically depressed or anxious. These rates were much higher than in other samples, with less-acculturated mothers having the highest rates. Particularly disturbing was that one-third had contemplated suicide in the past week. On a more hopeful note, the author noted that even with high levels of depression and anxiety, these mothers were still responsive to their babies (Foss, 2001).

POSTPARTUM PSYCHOSIS

Postpartum psychosis is the most serious form of postpartum mental illness. Although postpartum psychosis is not the focus of this book, it is important to mention because of its severity and its co-occurrence with depression. It occurs in 0.1 to 0.2 percent of all new mothers, and most episodes begin abruptly between three and fourteen days postpartum (Rapkin et al., 2002).

In two studies of women hospitalized for severe postpartum illness in Edinburgh, Scotland (Davidson & Robertson, 1985), and Kaduna, Nigeria (Ifabumuyi & Akindele, 1985), the three most common diagnoses were unipolar depression, bipolar depression, and schizophrenia. Transient organic psychosis was also a diagnosis for a small percentage of subjects in both studies.

More recently, Miller (2002) noted that the most common differential diagnoses for postpartum psychosis include major depression with psychotic features, bipolar disorder, schizoaffective disorder, schizophrenia, and brief reactive psychosis. Some medical conditions can be related to postpartum psychosis, and should be ruled out before diagnosing these symptoms as due to mood disorders. These other conditions include thyroiditis, hypothyroidism, vitamin B$_{12}$ deficiency, and adult GM2 gangliosidosis. Substances that can trigger a psychotic episode include bromocriptine, metronidazole, and addictive substances including LSD, PCP, and Ecstasy.

Bipolar Disorder

One type of postpartum psychosis is bipolar disorder. It is often overlooked because it usually manifests in the puerperium as major depression without psychosis. In a study of thirty bipolar women who had children, 66 percent had a postpartum episode of their illness (Freeman et al., 2002). Most of these episodes were exclusively depressive. Of the women who became depressed after their first child, all became depressed after subsequent births. Depression during any pregnancy also increased the risk of postpartum depression.

Birth can also trigger episodes of psychosis in bipolar women with a family history of postpartum psychosis (Jones & Craddock, 2001). One study examined 313 deliveries of 152 women with bipolar disorder. Twenty-six percent of the deliveries were followed by an episode of puerperal psychosis, and 38 percent of the women had at least one puerperal psychotic episode. Family history also increased risk. Of twenty-seven women with bipolar disorder who had a family history of postpartum psychosis, 74 percent developed postpartum psychosis. In contrast, only 30 percent of the women with bipolar disorder, but without a family history of postpartum psychosis, had a postpartum psychotic episode.

Women with bipolar disorder are often undiagnosed until after they have children (Freeman et al., 2002). However, they pose a treatment challenge. Since their illness often manifests as major depression in the postpartum period, they are often treated with selective serotonin reuptake inhibitors (SSRIs). Unfortunately, in women with bipolar disorder, these medications can also trigger manic or rapid-cycling episodes. For these women, the anticonvulsant medications may be more appropriate in that they have both mood-stabilizing and antidepressant effects (Leibenluft, 2000; see also Chapter 11).

CONDITIONS COMORBID
WITH POSTPARTUM DEPRESSION

Several conditions can co-occur with postpartum depression, including postpartum anxiety disorders, eating disorders, and substance abuse. These are described in the following sections.

Postpartum Anxiety Disorders

Postpartum anxiety disorders include panic disorders, generalized anxiety disorder, social phobia, obsessive-compulsive disorder (OCD), and post-traumatic stress disorder (PTSD). Several factors appear to contribute to postpartum anxiety disorders, including additional responsibilities and changing social, family, and professional roles (Rapkin et al., 2002).

In a community sample of 107 women, Stuart, Couser, Schilder, and O'Hara (1998) found that the point prevalence of postpartum anxiety was 9 percent at fourteen weeks, and 17 percent at thirty weeks postpartum. For depression, the point prevalence was 23 percent at fourteen weeks, and 19 percent at thirty weeks. They noted that higher percentages of women had either depression or anxiety in the postpartum period.

Cohen, Sichel, Dimmock, and Rosenbaum (1994) found that the impact of pregnancy on panic disorder was mixed. In this study, they retrospectively followed the clinical course of forty-nine women who had panic disorder before pregnancy and 78 percent of these women had either no change or a slight improvement while pregnant. For 27 percent of the women, their panic disorder became more severe during pregnancy. It appeared that patients with milder symptoms either improved or stayed the same during pregnancy. In contrast, women with more severe illness needed to continue treatment with antipanic medication during their pregnancies.

Obsessive-Compulsive Disorder

OCD is an anxiety disorder that often co-occurs with postpartum depression. It is characterized by recurrent, unwelcome thoughts, ideas, or doubts that give rise to anxiety and distress (obsessions). These obsessions lead to excessive behavioral or mental acts (Abramowitz, Schwartz, Moore, & Luenzmann, 2002). The exact incidence of postpartum OCD is not known, but birth of a child, particularly with high rates of obstetric complications, is one of the known triggers of symptoms (Maina, Albert, Bogetto, Vaschetto, & Ravizza, 1999).

In postpartum women, obsessional thoughts are often focused on infant harm. Some concern fears of harming the baby with knives, throwing the baby down stairs or out a window, or other types of harm (Abramowitz et al., 2002). Other types of compulsions concern mothers' repetitive thoughts of their babies dying in their sleep (e.g., sudden infant death syndrome [SIDS]), that they would sexually misuse their babies, or would physically misplace them. In a study of fifteen women with postpartum-onset OCD, all suffered from disabling intrusive obsessional thoughts of harming their babies. Most of these women were also depressed (Sichel, Cohen, Dimmock, & Rosenbaum, 1993). Not surprisingly, obsessive thoughts can be very troubling to mothers, as DeeDee describes.

My postpartum depression was basically weird thoughts toward the baby, and he was a wonderful baby. The perfect baby. One time I had him on the bathroom floor with me. All of the sudden, I had this thought to kick the baby. This was the first weird thought I had toward him. My pediatrician told me that this was very normal. "You had a traumatic delivery." . . . I would have weird thoughts when I was breastfeeding. I was constantly worried that the baby would hit his head on the table. I was also scared to walk through the doorway, that he would hit his head. These thoughts would become obsessive. I was afraid if I told anyone, they'd take the baby away. I finally told my mom. She said it was normal and not to worry. This lasted around five months. . . . If I was ironing, I'd be terrified that the baby would be burned. Even if he was upstairs asleep in his bed. Then I would start to analyze my thoughts. "Am I thinking he'd be burned because I wanted him to be burned?" I was also scared of knives. . . . I didn't want to do these things. I couldn't understand why I was thinking this way. . . . These thoughts happened every day, all the time. Slowly, I had fewer thoughts. I'd think, "There's no way he can hit his head when I'm holding him." . . . The hardest thing was, I couldn't find anyone who had this experience. I knew about it, but I couldn't seem to find anyone who had been through it.

Wisner, Peindl, Gigliotti, and Hanusa (1999) compared women with postpartum depression and women with nonpostpartum depression. In both these groups, high rates of OCD co-occurred with depression. Fifty-seven percent of the postpartum women had OCD symptoms, as did 36 percent of the nonpostpartum depressed women. This difference between the groups was not significant. The authors concluded that childbearing women are more likely to experience obsessional thoughts and compulsions when experiencing major depression. In another study, 29 percent of women with preexisting OCD reported an exacerbation of their symptoms in the postpartum period and 37 percent reported depression (Williams & Koran, 1997).

A study of four men revealed that they too experienced postpartum OCD that coincided with their wives' deliveries. These obsessions were very similar in content to the obsessional thoughts of new mothers. The men responded with feelings of shame and guilt (Abramowitz, Moore, Carmin, Wiegartz, & Purdon, 2001).

Beck (2002) identified anxiety, relentless obsessive thinking, anger, guilt, and contemplating self-harm as part of her "spiraling down" dimension of postpartum depression. This dimension was part of a metasynthesis of eighteen qualitative studies of postpartum depression. Obsessive thoughts were so intrusive for the women in Beck's (1993, 2002) studies that they often became intolerable. Women tended to ruminate over feelings of failure as a mother, fearing that they or their babies might be harmed, wondering if they would ever feel normal again, and constantly worrying about the baby. These mothers tended to self-silence and isolate themselves because they were sure no one would understand what they were going through.

Responding to concerns about infant harm. Descriptions of thoughts about harming the baby must also be handled with great care. Women I have spoken with indicated that professionals either reacted with great alarm or assured them that the thoughts were "normal." The women who were troubled by these thoughts indicated that one of the worst reactions people had was to become alarmed and express great concern that they would kill their babies. This reaction did not stop the thoughts but actually fed into them and made them more intense.

Abramowitz et al., (2002) distinguish obsessive thoughts of infant harm from psychosis. In psychosis, thoughts of harm are consistent with a person's delusional thinking. A person acts out aggressively because she believes she has to do it. In contrast, obsessive thoughts do not increase risk of infant harm. These thoughts are unwanted and inconsistent with a person's normal behavior and are so distressing that people suffering from OCD will go to great lengths to prevent these bad things from happening.

It is also unhelpful when professionals dismiss these thoughts as normal because the women themselves know that they are not. They may be fairly commonplace, but that does not mean they are normal. When speaking to a mother, you can say something like this: "It must be very distressing to you to have such thoughts. Many other women have these thoughts, and they do not mean that you are a bad mother or will harm your baby. These thoughts usually mean that you are under some type of stress, and it may help to talk with someone about it." Then you can offer some names of people who can help. This type of approach validates a woman's experience while taking the problem seriously.

In more serious cases, you may need to take additional action. If the mother refuses help, or if you fear that the baby is in danger, you may be legally obligated to make a report to the department of social services or your local child protective agency.

Post-Traumatic Stress Disorder

Another co-occurring anxiety disorder is PTSD. Women may come into the postpartum period with preexisting vulnerability to PTSD. PTSD could be due to prior trauma, such as previous abuse or sexual assault, or it could be caused by the birth itself. Even if women do not meet full criteria for PTSD, they may have troubling symptoms. In the study of Vietnamese and Hmong women described earlier, Foss (2001) found that PTSD was highly correlated with depression in this sample. PTSD in postpartum women is described more fully in Chapter 4.

Eating Disorders

Eating disorders can also co-occur with depression during pregnancy and the postpartum period. In a sample of forty-nine women with eating disorders who had recently given birth, the rate of postpartum depression was 35 percent (Franko et al., 2001). The majority of these women had normal pregnancies, but three women had babies with birth defects. Among the women in the study, those who had active symptoms of either anorexia or bulimia during pregnancy were at increased risk for postpartum depression. The authors recommended close monitoring of women with past or current eating disorders during pregnancy and in the postpartum period.

In a study of 181 women, binge eating and vomiting before pregnancy predicted postpartum depression. Mothers whose eating disorders were active during pregnancy were the most distressed in this sample, particularly those with a binge or purge type of eating disorder. However, low-intensity exercise was associated with less distress (Abraham, Taylor, & Conti, 2001).

Eating disorders were also associated with the discipline style mothers chose to use. Mothers with eating disorders were more likely to employ verbal control, especially strong control, as a form of discipline with their one-year-olds than mothers with postpartum depression or a healthy comparison group (Stein et al., 2001).

Substance Abuse

Finally, substance abuse can also co-occur with postpartum depression. Two studies have considered the link between substance abuse and depression in mothers. In the first study (Pajulo, Savonlahti, Sourander, Helenius, & Piha, 2001), 8 percent of 391 pregnant women were depressed. Substance abuse and life stress both predicted depression in pregnancy, as did difficulties with their social networks (friends, partners, and the women's own mothers).

A second study (Pajulo, Savonlahti, Sourander, Ahlqvist, et al., 2001) compared twelve mothers who abused substances and twelve control mothers in their emotional health and interactions with their babies at three and six months postpartum. Not surprisingly, the substance-abusing mothers were significantly more depressed, had less social support, and had more life stress than the control mothers. Their interactions with their babies were also less positive.

Substance abuse is obviously a serious problem for both mothers and babies. If a woman abuses substances during pregnancy, the state may intervene and remove the baby from her care after delivery. For substance-abusing mothers, intervention for depression alone would be incomplete. Mothers who abuse substances also need referrals to programs that can directly address substance abuse.

CONCLUSION

Postpartum depression is responsible for a wide range of symptoms and can co-occur with other conditions such as anxiety disorders, eating disorders, and substance abuse. Bipolar disorder can also appear in the postpartum period and may manifest as major depression or postpartum psychosis. In the next chapter, I describe why depression is harmful for mothers and babies.

Chapter 2

Why Depression Is Harmful for Mothers and Babies

Depression is bad for mothers and babies. And it is expensive. In a study of 6,000 primary care patients, depressed patients had significantly higher health care costs of all types, including specialty, inpatient, pharmacy, and laboratory, than patients who were not depressed. The elevated costs remained even after the patients were no longer depressed (Simon, Ormel, VonKorff, & Barlow, 1995). In a ten-year longitudinal study, depressive symptoms were associated with increased outpatient visits, even when patients were no longer depressed, and even after controlling for age, sex, marital status, medical comorbidity, and patient status (Kimberling, Ouimette, Cronkite, & Moos, 1999).

Findings with populations of new mothers have been similar. In a Canadian study (Roberts et al., 2001), maternal depression was one of the five factors significantly associated with higher nursing costs for postpartum families. The other factors included mothers with more than five learning needs, mother's perceived poor health, mother's perceived lack of help and support at home, and a postpartum stay of less than forty-eight hours. Depressed mothers had health care costs that were twice those of nondepressed mothers, and very depressed mothers had costs that were five times higher.

These studies demonstrate that depression is costly and it also has a negative impact on health of mothers and babies. This research is summarized in this chapter.

WHY DEPRESSION IS BAD FOR MOTHERS

Depression has a profound and devastating impact on the health of mothers. In the Global Burden of Disease Study, major depression was the fourth most common cause of early death and disability throughout the world, and second only to coronary artery disease in industrialized countries (Murray & Lopez, 1997).

Some of the health problems associated with depression are due to the stress hormone cortisol, which is often elevated in people who are depressed. Elevated levels of cortisol can suppress the immune system, cause cardiovascular dysfunctions, and even lower the number of white blood cells (Campeau, Day, Helmreich, Kollack-Walker, & Walker, 1998). Increased levels of cortisol can also lead to atrophy of the hippocampus, a brain structure involved in learning and memory. Depressed patients, even formerly depressed patients, had a lower hippocampal volume than patients who were not depressed. The decrease in volume ranged from 12 percent in the right hippocampus to 19 percent in the left hippocampus (Sapolsky, 2000).

Depression and Cardiovascular Health

Depression has been related to cardiovascular disease in several studies (Remick, 2002). For example, in a large study of patients (N = 1,551) without heart disease, an episode of major depression increased the risk of heart attack 4.5 times (Pratt et al., 1996). This risk was independent of other risk factors including age, ventricular ejection fraction, and diabetes mellitus.

According to one review, patients who became depressed after a myocardial infarction were three to four times more likely to die than those who were not depressed (Lesperance & Frasure-Smith, 2000). The risk existed not only for those suffering from major depression but also for those having milder forms as well. Cardiovascular events are less likely in a population of new mothers, but these studies illustrate depression's serious health effects.

Depression and Immune System Function

Depression can also suppress the immune system, working directly on the white blood cells (Avissar, Nechamkin, Roitman, & Schreiber, 1997; Weisse, 1992). For example, in a sample of HIV-positive men, depression was associated with fewer CD4 T lymphocytes and lower proliferative responses to the mitogen phytohemagglutinin (Kemeny, Weiner, Taylor, & Schneider, 1994). Another prospective study of HIV-positive men had similar findings (Leserman et al., 1997). In this study, severe stress and depression were related to decreases in immune function from study entry to a follow-up two years later. Specifically, the authors noted declines in CD8+ T cells and CD56+ and CD 16+ NK cell subsets. They concluded that since these cells are important in terms of maintaining health, suppression of these cells had clinical implications for progression of HIV.

High levels of perceived stress led to significantly lower levels of two cytokines—interleukin 1 (alpha) and interleukin 8. From a biochemical standpoint, severe stress and depression show a similar pattern. These same subjects had higher salivary cortisol levels than those who had high cytokine levels (Glaser et al., 1999). So while these cytokines might be initially elevated in people who are depressed, the high levels trigger the release of cortisol to get the cytokines under control. Cortisol then suppresses and inhibits immune function.

Depression and Health Behaviors

Depression is also related to health behaviors. In a review of the literature, negative emotions were correlated with poor eating habits, use of tobacco, and abuse of alcohol and drugs. People may use these harmful behaviors as a way to cope with negative emotions. Even chocolate consumption increases when people are depressed (Salovey, Rothman, Detweiler, & Steward, 2000).

In a study of more than 5,000 male and female college students, depression was associated with lack of physical activity, not eating breakfast, irregular sleep hours, and not using a seat belt in men and women. In addition, depression was associated with smoking, not eating fruit, and not using sunscreen in women (Allgower, Wardle, & Steptoe, 2001).

So we see that depression has serious health implications for mothers, including increased risk of cardiovascular diseases, a suppressed immune system, and decreased health behaviors. However, depression in mothers is also harmful to babies.

WHY DEPRESSION IN MOTHERS IS BAD FOR BABIES

A wealth of studies over the past twenty years has demonstrated the harmful effects of maternal depression on children. These studies run the gamut from the neonatal period to young adulthood. Following is a summary of these findings.

Effects on Infants

Depression during pregnancy can lead to elevations of stress hormones in neonates. In one study, sixty-three mothers were recruited during the last trimester of pregnancy, thirty-six of whom had depressive symptoms. Their infants were tested in the first seven days of life. The depressed women and their babies had higher cortisol and norepinephrine levels and lower dopamine levels. These neonates also performed more poorly on the orientation, reflex, excitability, and withdrawal clusters of the Brazelton Neonatal Behavioral Assessment Scale (Lundy, Jones, Field, & Nearing, 1999).

Abnormalities in electroencephalograms (EEGs) have also been observed in infants at three to six months. The sample was thirty-two mothers who were all low-income, single, adolescents of African American or Hispanic ethnicity. The babies were all full term with no medical conditions. These babies showed depressed affect and had right frontal EEG asymmetry as early as three months (Field, Fox, Pickens, & Nawrocki, 1995). This is an abnormal pattern found in chronically depressed adults. Another study of forty-eight neonates (Field, Diego, Hernandez-Reif, Schanberg, & Kuhn, 2002) found that babies with greater relative right frontal EEG had elevated cortisol levels, showed more variability in state changes during sleep/wake observations, and had less than optimum performance on the Brazelton Neonatal Behavior Assessment Scale. Their mothers also had lower prenatal and postnatal serotonin levels and higher levels of cortisol (both suggesting depression). The authors concluded that greater relative right frontal activation may place these infants at greater risk for developmental problems.

Another study (Whiffen & Gotlib, 1989) compared twenty-five depressed and twenty-five nondepressed mothers of two-month-olds. Infants of depressed mothers performed significantly more poorly on the Bayley Scales of Infant Development and expressed more negative emotions during testing. The infants of depressed mothers were more tense, less content, deteriorated more quickly under testing, and became more distressed as testing continued. The authors concluded that these infants responded more quickly to stress and that this could be due to a dysfunctional relationship between mother and baby. They also speculated that depressed mothers were less efficient at working their schedules, so that babies might be exposed to more stressors, such as delayed feedings or diaper changes. Therefore, these mothers saw more negative behaviors from their babies as they expressed their distress. The depressed mothers also perceived their infants as more difficult to care for, but they were more likely to blame themselves rather than their babies for any difficulties they encountered.

In Barbados, in a sample of 226 mother-infant pairs, maternal depression at seven weeks postpartum predicted lower infant social and performance scores at three months. Depression at six months was associated with lower infant scores in motor development at the same age (Galler, Harrison, Ramsey, Forde, & Butler, 2000).

Effects on Preschoolers

Maternal depression can also affect preschoolers. In a community sample of 119 primiparous women, children of mothers with post-partum depression had lower scores on the McCarthy Scales of Children's Abilities at age four years. The McCarthy scales are a measure of overall intelligence. Perceptual performance was most adversely affected. These findings were not accounted for by prenatal and perinatal experiences, nor the family's current status. Low birth weight enhanced the negative effect of maternal depression on these children. But the effect of depression was lessened for mothers who had higher levels of education (Hay & Kumar, 1995).

In another study of four- to five-year-olds born to adolescent mothers, Black and colleagues (2002) found that maternal depression and the mother's perceptions of her partner influenced children's behavior problems. This was a high-risk sample; 42.4 percent of the children had been maltreated, 36 percent had externalizing scores in the clinical range, and 10.8 percent had internalizing scores in the clinical range. In this study, maternal depression was the mechanism underlying the link between mother's perception of quality of the partner relationship and children's behavior problems (especially internalizing). When mothers were depressed, the perceived quality of their relationship with their partner became worse and their children showed more symptoms.

Effects on School-Age Children

The negative impact of maternal depression can last into elementary school. In an American study of 5,000 mother-infant pairs, children of depressed mothers had more behavior problems and lower vocabulary scores at age five (Brennan et al., 2000). In this study, mothers were assessed for depression during pregnancy, immediately postpartum, and when the child was six months and five years old. Severity and chronicity of depression were related to more behavior problems, as were more recent episodes of depression.

Murray, Woolgar, Cooper, and Hipwell (2001) found that children of depressed mothers were more likely, at age five, to express depressive cognitions such as hopelessness, pessimism, and low self-worth, especially when exposed to a mild stressor. The authors noted, however, that much of this relationship can be accounted for by current maternal hostility toward the child. In another study, maternal depression during the child's first two years of life was the best predictor of elevations in baseline cortisol in response to a mild stressor at age seven (Ashman, Dawson, Panagiotides, Yamada, & Wilkins, 2002).

Children of mothers who had postpartum depression were lower in social competence at ages eight to nine in a study from Finland (Luoma et al., 2001). Social competence included parents' reports of children's activities, hobbies, tasks, and chores; functioning in social relationships; and school achievements. Mothers were assessed for depression prenatally, postnatally, and when their children were eight to nine years old. Mothers' current depression was also associated with low social competence and low adaptive functioning.

Negative findings also appear at age eleven (Hay et al., 2001). In this study, women were assessed for depression at three months postpartum (N = 149). At age eleven, 132 of these children were tested. Children of mothers who were depressed at three months postpartum had significantly lower IQ scores and had a number of problems in school, including attentional problems and difficulties in mathematical reasoning. They were more likely to be in special education. The effects were particularly pronounced for boys. The links between postpartum depression and IQ were not accounted for by social disadvantage or by mothers' later mental health problems.

Effects on Young Adults

The lifetime risk of depression is also increased well into adulthood. In a study of 2,427 young adults (Lieb, Isensee, Hofler, Pfister, & Wittchen, 2002), depression in either their mothers or fathers increased the risk of depression in the subjects. Interestingly, paternal depression was associated with an earlier onset of depression and increased severity, impairment, and recurrence in their children.

Maternal Depression and Infant Health Behaviors

As was found in regard to depression and self-care, depression has also been shown to have a negative impact on parent-based prevention practices in one study. In this study (McLennan & Kotelchuck, 2000), 7,537 mothers with newborns were surveyed in 1988 and then contacted again in 1991. The authors found that mothers with high levels of depression reported significantly poorer prevention practices for infant safety. These practices included car seat use, covering electrical plugs, and having syrup of ipecac in the home.

Similarly, in a large, national, representative sample, Leiferman (2002) found that depressed mothers were more likely to smoke. They were less likely to administer vitamins to their two- to four-year-olds and were less likely to use car seats or restrain their children properly in the car.

Depression also influenced breastfeeding. In a study from Barbados, mothers depressed at seven weeks were less interested in breastfeeding at current and later infant ages. In that culture, the cessation of breastfeeding could influence infant survival, especially since the depressed mothers also had lower family income, poor maternal health, and lower levels of information seeking by the mother (Galler, Harrison, Biggs, Ramsey, & Forde, 1999).

INTERACTION STYLES OF DEPRESSED MOTHERS

Depression in mothers can lead to some long-lasting and serious effects in their babies. The next logical question is to ask why this occurs. To understand why, it is instructive to look at the interaction styles of depressed mothers. In general, we know that depressed mothers generally show flat affect with their babies. They provide less stimulation to their babies and less contingent responsivity. The babies are less attentive, have fewer contented expressions, are fussier, and have lower activity levels.

Depression can also influence women's feelings about interacting with their babies. In one study, depressed women were more likely to describe their infants as difficult to care for at two months postpartum and to indicate that they felt overwhelmed by child care than were their nondepressed counterparts (Campbell, Cohn, Flanagan, Popper, & Meyers, 1992). In another study, depressed women expressed fewer positive emotions with their infants, were less expressive or involved, and were less responsive or sensitive to their babies' needs than were the nondepressed women (Hoffman & Drotar, 1991).

In a study of 570 Swiss three-month-olds (Righetti-Veltema, Conne-Perreard, Bousquet, & Manzano, 2002), depressed mother-infant dyads showed less vocal or visual communication, had less corporal interaction, and smiled less than their nondepressed counterparts. In another study, mothers were assessed for depression at two months postpartum and were filmed interacting with their babies at fifteen to eighteen months postpartum. Children of depressed women showed fewer attention skills in free play and were more likely to have an insecure attachment, or a secure attachment with "restricted joy" (Edhborg, Lundh, Seimyr, & Widstroem, 2001).

In a meta-analysis of nineteen studies, Beck (1995) found that depression had a moderate to large effect on infants. Depressed women were less likely to display affectionate contact behavior with their babies and were less responsive to their infants or their infants' cues. In another study (Albertsson-Karlgren, Graff, & Nettelbladt, 2001), women who had mental illness (including depression and psychosis) were videotaped with their infants at ten months postpartum. These mothers showed less sensitivity than comparison mothers who were being treated for physical health problems. When the infants were two years old, the mothers in the psychiatric group also showed less positive affect than the mothers with physical health problems.

Beyond these general behaviors, depressed mothers tend to fall into two basic interaction styles. These are described in the following section.

Avoidant and Angry-Intrusive Interaction Styles

Depressed mothers tend to have one of two basic interaction styles: avoidant and angry-intrusive (Beck, 1995; Field, 1992; Tronick & Weinberg, 1997). In the avoidant style, mothers spend approximately 80 percent of their time disengaged from their babies, ignoring their cues. Mothers with this style are unresponsive, have flat affect, and do not support their infants' activities; they only respond to infant distress. Babies react to this style by trying to engage their mothers in interaction. Unfortunately, they are generally not successful. This lack of maternal responsiveness is highly stressful for babies, as demonstrated by elevated cortisol levels and abnormal EEG patterns. These infants protest about 30 percent of the time and watch their mothers less than 5 percent of the time. They become disengaged, and engage in self-comforting, self-regulatory behaviors such as thumb sucking, looking away, passivity, and withdrawal to help them cope with their state. When they cannot engage their mothers, they often respond by "shutting down" (Field, 1992).

In the angry-intrusive style, mothers are more engaged with their babies, but the interactions are characterized by hostility and intrusiveness. In this style, mothers express anger and irritation and handle their babies roughly approximately 40 percent of the time. These mothers also ignore their babies' cues. Mothers with the angry/intrusive style speak in an angry tone, poke at their babies, and interfere with their babies' activities (Tronick & Weinberg, 1997). Rather than interacting in a give-and-take fashion, these mothers dominate the relationship. It does not matter what the baby wants or needs at a particular moment. Babies react to this style by trying to disengage from their mothers approximately 55 percent of the time (e.g., arching or looking or pushing away). They only protest about 5 percent of the time. These infants are often angry and show frustration easily in anticipation of their mothers' intrusiveness (Tronick & Weinberg, 1997). Mothers may interpret this behavior as rejection (Field, 1992).

In Beck's (1996b) phenomenological study of twelve mothers with postpartum depression, mothers reported on their subjective experiences. The themes of both anger and avoidance are woven throughout these accounts. In this sample, participants indicated that they were overwhelmed by their child care responsibilities. Their day-to-day interactions with their children were filled with guilt, irrational thinking, loss, and anger. The mothers reported that they went through their days "like robots," simply going through the motions. They also responded to the overwhelming needs of their babies by building walls to separate themselves emotionally from them. Eventually, their interactions with their babies spilled over and influenced their interactions with their older children as well. One mother, who was experiencing detachment from her baby, reported, "The baby would be on the table looking at me, dressed, washed, looking at me, cooing and laughing and smiling, and I just looked at her" (Beck, 1996b, p. 100). Another mother reported how depression made her feel extremely angry:

> I felt so much anger inside of me. I had to stop and think that this little baby doesn't know any better. I looked up and saw my husband in the doorway, and I said, "Get the baby away!" (Beck, 1996b, p. 100)

When interacting with their mothers, infants of depressed mothers were fussier, more discontented, more avoidant, and were less likely to make positive facial expressions and vocalizations than infants of nondepressed mothers. They also showed elevated heart rates and cortisol levels. These signs indicated that the interactions were stressful for the babies. The mother-infant dyads also had difficulty matching their behavioral states to each other and synchronizing their interactions with each other (Field, 1995). Not only that, but regardless of the mother's interaction style, these infants invariably appeared depressed, and they tended to elicit depression-like interactions from others (Field, 1992). For indications of healthy mother-infant interaction see Exhibit 2.1.

The Still-Faced Mother Studies

The still-faced mother paradigm has been used in many studies to demonstrate—under laboratory conditions—the effects of maternal depression. Mothers were asked to pretend that they were depressed when interacting with their three-month-old babies (Weinberg & Tronick, 1998; Moore et al., 2001). These mothers spoke in a monotone, had little or no facial affect, and hardly touched their infants. It only took about three minutes before the infants became distressed at the way their mothers were acting. The infants became wary and tried

EXHIBIT 2.1. Characteristics of Positive Mother-Infant Interaction

An effective (or synchronous) mother-child interaction contains many components (Capuzzi, 1989). The mother and infant must give clear cues to each other; the mother must be responsive to the infant's cues; the infant must respond to the mother's caregiving; and the environment must be supportive of and facilitate this interaction. This is the process by which mothers become attached to their infants. When this process breaks down, it can lead to insecure attachments between mothers and babies, and maternal depression.

to engage their mothers in their normal affective states. The infants continued to be wary even when mothers returned to their normal affect (Weinberg & Tronick, 1998). This paradigm was designed to assess infants' reactions to a break in normal social interaction. Infants often responded by trying to elicit responses from their mothers by smiling briefly. However, when their mothers did not respond, the infants became distressed (Moore, Cohn, & Campbell, 2001).

One study also tried to determine whether reactions to the still-face predicted problems in later development for infants of depressed and nondepressed mothers. In this study, 129 mother-infant pairs participated. Approximately half of the mothers met criteria for major depressive disorder. The infants were assessed at two, four, and six months (Moore et al., 2001). The infants' responses predicted internalizing and externalizing behaviors at eighteen months. Moore et al.'s findings demonstrated that infants are sensitive to disruptions in social reciprocity as early as two months of age.

Intervention for Depressed Mothers

If the interaction of depressed mothers is dysfunctional, does it improve when depression resolves? Conversely, does depression remit when the interaction improves? The findings have been mixed. In a study of 117 postpartum women with depressive symptoms (Horowitz et al., 2001), half of the women were assigned to a treatment group in which they were coached to improve in their responsiveness to their infants. At the end of the intervention, mothers in the intervention group did show significantly higher levels of maternal responsiveness, but the intervention had no effect on their symptoms of depression.

Armstrong, Fraser, Dadds, and Morris (1999), in a double-blind controlled study, found that a home visiting program that helped mothers develop secure attachments to their babies decreased depression at six weeks. Similarly, Field (1997) reviewed the literature on interventions for depressed mothers and found that techniques such as massage for the mothers, and teaching the mothers infant massage, lowered stress hormones for both. Teaching mothers infant massage also makes mothers more in tune with their babies' cues.

According to a review (McLennan & Offord, 2002), it is unclear whether targeting postpartum depression alone is enough to ameliorate these negative child outcomes. Depression and negative interaction style may need to be addressed separately. In the next section I describe two of the most serious and disturbing forms of mother and infant harm.

INFANTICIDE AND MATERNAL SUICIDE

Perhaps the most shocking reaction to postpartum illness is when a mother takes her own life or that of her baby. Scott (1987) characterized these responses as the "extreme tip of the iceberg" in terms of puerperal depression. Unfortunately, we know very little about this from scientific inquiry. Most of what we know is based on anecdotal evidence and clinical reports. Nevertheless, these anecdotal reports do shed some light on this frightening response.

Davidson and Robertson (1985) conducted one of the earliest empirical studies of infanticide and suicide in puerperal women. They followed eighty-two patients who had been hospitalized for postpartum illness between 1946 and 1971. Of these eighty-two women with severe postpartum reactions, 52 percent were diagnosed with unipolar depression, 18 percent with bipolar depression, 16 percent with schizophrenia, and 11 percent with other mental illnesses. Of this group, 5 percent ultimately committed suicide, and approximately 4 percent had committed infanticide (some of the cases had not been confirmed). Of the patients that committed suicide, two had unipolar depression and two were schizophrenic. Only one of the suicides occurred during the postpartum period. One took place after three years, and the other two took place after twelve years. One woman with unipolar depression was known to have committed infanticide, and another was strongly suspected to have done so. One of the women with schizophrenia killed her two youngest children at eighteen months postpartum.

Infanticide

Chandra, Vankatasubramanian, and Thomas (2002) studied fifty Indian women who had been admitted to a psychiatric hospital postpartum. They collected data from three sources: from the mother's partner, from nursing observations made during the first week in the hospital, and from the psychiatric assessment within the first week of admission. In this sample, 43 percent reported infanticidal ideas, 36 percent reported infanticidal behavior, and 34 percent reported both infanticidal ideas and behavior. Infanticidal ideas and behavior tended to co-occur. In a logistic regression, depression and psychotic ideas predicted infanticidal ideas. Psychotic ideas also predicted infanticidal behavior.

A study from Finland (Haapasalo & Petaja, 1999) examined mental state examination reports from forty-eight mothers who killed or attempted to kill their children. In this study, they differentiated between neonaticides (within the first twenty-four hours) and subsequent deaths for children under the age of twelve. The majority of these nonneonatal killings were children under the age of four ($N = 33$). The nonneonaticide killings are of most interest to our present discussion. The women who killed their babies in the first twenty-four hours tended to be young, unmarried women who denied that they were pregnant. In contrast, the nonneonatal killings were committed by married women, living with a spouse, and who were significantly more likely to be homemakers. Two-thirds of these women had documented psychological problems, including depression (81 percent), anxiety and fear (45 percent), psychosis (30 percent), and somatization and eating disorders (27 percent). Only 9 percent had obsessional thoughts. Sixty-three percent of these mothers had a history of some form of child maltreatment. The most common was psychological abuse (44 percent), followed by physical abuse (25 percent), neglect (10 percent), and sexual abuse (6 percent). Only 15 percent of these killings were due to postpartum depression. The others were joint suicide-homicide attempts, impulsive aggression, psychotic episodes, and abusive acts. Before the homicides, most of these mothers were reported to be "perfect" mothers who had taken good care of their children.

Case Studies

Andrea Yates is perhaps the most well known of women who have killed children as a result of postpartum mental illness. Mrs. Yates systematically drowned her five children, laid their bodies out on the bed, and then called her husband to tell him what she had done. According to her psychiatrist, she was suffering from schizophrenia and major depression. These conditions impaired her thinking and resulted in delusions, hallucinations, and social withdrawal. Her condition first surfaced after the birth of her fourth child in 1999. She attempted suicide twice that year, and she and her husband were cautioned not to have any more children. After her fifth child's birth in 2000, the delusions and voices become more intense (Charatan, 2002).

Psychotic beliefs were very much part of the motivation for Andrea Yates to drown her five children. Three weeks after she killed her children, she explained that Satan was telling her that she was such a bad mother that she had to kill her children to keep them from going to hell. She indicated that the state would execute her, and that would eliminate Satan from the world, and that she could save her children by killing them. God would "take them up" (Charatan, 2002, p. 2). In 2003, Texas passed an "Andrea Yates bill" that requires all obstetricians, midwives, birthing centers, and hospitals to provide pregnant women with a list of professional organizations that can help with postpartum depression. Ironically, the law named after her probably would not have helped Andrea Yates. Her postpartum depression had already been identified, and she was in treatment when she had her psychotic episode.

These types of delusions were also recorded in other publicized cases of infanticide. For example, Angela Thompson became delusional after she stopped breastfeeding her son at age nine months. She drowned him in the bathtub after hearing the voice of God tell her the child was the devil (Toufexis, 1988). Sheryl Massip heard voices that compelled her to kill her six-week-old son. She finally did when she ran over him with her car (Meyer & Oberman, 2001).

In other cases, the link between infanticide and postpartum illness is less clear. For example, Lucrezia Gentile drowned her two-month-old son because she could not stand his incessant crying. Kathleen Householder hit her two-week-old daughter with a rock because she was fussing (Toufexis, 1988). Michele Remington shot her infant son before she tried to take her own life. These cases appear to be fatal child abuse rather than reactions to postpartum illness. But it is often difficult to tell. Meyer and Oberman (2001), in their book on mothers who kill their children, noted that in the case of infanticide it is often difficult to distinguish "mad" from "bad." Elements of both are often present. In some cases, there are clear indications of postpartum psychosis, such as delusional thinking. But other cases often involve pre-existing life stresses, such as past or current abuse, substance abuse, or some other impairing factor.

Maternal Suicide

Maternal suicide is another startling and tragic reaction to postpartum illness. It is often even more difficult to establish a link between postpartum illness and suicide since it might not occur until several months after a woman has a baby. In one case, Victoria Karter, age thirty-three, checked into the Four Seasons Hotel and jumped to her death five months after the birth of her daughter (Kalfus & Shaffer, 1990). To outside observers, Mrs. Karter had a complete and happy life: stable marital relationship, good relationship with her family, and beautiful new baby. But Mrs. Karter's depression had been increasingly severe over the previous several months, and she had been in treatment for postpartum depression prior to her death.

A study of maternal deaths in Sweden from 1980 to 1988 found a total number of fifty-eight early maternal deaths. Suicide was the cause in 10 percent (Hogberg, Innala, & Sandstrom, 1994). Similarly, in a study of twenty-two consecutive maternal deaths in Australia, two of the deaths (11 percent) were suicides at three and four months postpartum (Henry, Sheedy, & Beischer, 1989). Of the seventy-six late maternal deaths (occurring from 43 to 365 days postpartum), suicide was identified as a "major cause," behind malignancy, stroke, and heart disease (Hogberg et al., 1994).

In a study from the Danish Psychiatric Case Register and the Danish registers of birth and causes of death (1973 to 1993), a total of

1,567 women had been admitted to psychiatric hospitals during the postpartum period. Of these women, 107 (6.8 percent) had died. The authors concluded that suicide risk among the general population of postpartum women is low. However, among the population of hospitalized postpartum women, the risk of suicide is high, especially in the first postpartum year when suicide risk is increased seventyfold (Appleby, Mortensen, & Faragher, 1998).

Suicide is relatively rare. However, as with thoughts of harming the baby, we do not know the incidence or prevalence of suicidal ideation. In a sample of hospitalized women in Australia (Fisher, Feekery, & Rowe-Murray, 2002), 5 percent reported suicidal ideation. Four mothers I have spoken with indicated that they had these types of thoughts.

I'm still dealing with the sexual abuse [her own past history]. I hadn't dealt with it before the birth. I told my husband [for the first time] in the hospital. I was hysterical. . . . I was afraid of being alone so my husband stayed the night. If I could've opened the window, I would have jumped out. (Val)

I had breastfeeding problems. He was colicky. I was afraid I wouldn't be able to comfort him. I didn't have thoughts of hurting him, but I thought of suicide. That's how depressed I was. (Elizabeth)

The severe depression would come on and go away. One time I was sorting through all our medicines, sorting the ones that were very lethal into a pile. The severe episodes only lasted about one to two minutes, but the moderate depression stayed. I couldn't be left alone. (Melissa)

My husband and sister thought they would take care of me. I started having visions of my own funeral. I was having all kinds of scary thoughts. At that point, they decided I needed to go into the hospital. . . . The week after my daughter's birthday, I was acutely suicidal. I packed some clothes and my pills. I was going to go to New York City, rent a hotel room, and kill myself. My husband said I was rambling and saying please take care of her. As I was getting on the train, my husband was at the train station because they found my car. (Dawn)

Obviously, any mention of suicide needs to be taken seriously. In most cases, mothers will not make a suicide attempt. But it is obviously better to be safe than sorry. In Chapter 8, I describe some general screening questions for suicide risk and need for hospitalization. Care must also be used in medication choice for mothers at risk for suicide. Safer choices for suicidal mothers are described in Chapter 11.

CONCLUSION

Depression causes more harm to mother and baby than people generally realize. These effects provide ample reason to take depression seriously and encourage mothers to seek treatment. In working with mothers, however, you must be careful in how you handle the information about infant harm. Although it can be helpful in motivating women to seek services, we must never communicate that their depression has somehow "ruined" their babies or children. Many times, mothers fear this, and this belief has been a motivating factor in some cases of infanticide. We can use this information to gently encourage mothers to get help because when they get better, it will also be good for their babies.

Now that we know of the seriousness of depression for mothers and babies, it makes sense to consider the risk factors for it. In the next five chapters I describe some of the risk factors associated with postpartum depression. Each of these risk factors offers opportunities for intervention.

Chapter 3

Physiological Influences in Postpartum Depression

A large number of physiological factors are related to postpartum depression. These include fatigue, hypothyroidism, pain, immune system responses, and even cholesterol levels. In this chapter, I describe what we know, so far, about the physiological underpinnings of postpartum depression.

FATIGUE AND SLEEP DEPRIVATION

Fatigue can be both a symptom of depression and a cause. The relationship between fatigue and depression is often a chicken-and-egg type of question. We do not know which came first. But fatigue can be a clue that something is amiss, particularly when women cannot sleep even when their babies are sleeping. Fatigue may be the way that depression presents. This is especially true in developing countries or in subcultures in the United States in which presenting a physical problem may be more culturally acceptable than saying you are depressed (Patel, Abas, Broadhead, Todd, & Reeler, 2001).

Fatigue's role in postpartum depression is often overlooked because almost all new mothers are tired (Bozoky & Corwin, 2002). One large Australian study found that 60 percent of new mothers reported exhaustion or extreme tiredness, and 30 percent reported lack of sleep due to their baby's crying in the first eight weeks (Thompson, Roberts, Currie, & Ellwood, 2002). These problems eventually resolved, but 49 percent still reported exhaustion, and 15 percent reported lack of sleep at twenty-four weeks. Mothers who had cesarean sections were more likely to report exhaustion than mothers with assisted or unassisted vaginal deliveries.

Fatigue is even more prominent in women with postpartum depression. In a sample of 109 women who were hospitalized in a mother-baby psychiatric unit, 91 percent of the women were clinically fatigued (Fisher, Feekery, & Rowe-Murray, 2002). These mothers also felt overwhelmed (76 percent) and anxious (75 percent). Some things that distinguished hospitalized women from postpartum women in general were a greater number of obstetric and reproductive problems, poor postpartum hospital care, lack of social connections, partners who worked long hours, inadequate practical assistance, and the presence of other stressful life events.

Severe fatigue also predicts future depression. One study recruited thirty-eight healthy new mothers who had uncomplicated births in the first day postpartum (Bozoky & Corwin, 2002). The author assessed fatigue on days 0, 7, 14, and 28 postpartum, and depression at day 28. They found that fatigue at day 7 predicted depression at day 28. Indeed, fatigue on day 7 accounted for 21 percent of the variance in depressive symptoms. Fatigue was not related to marital status, presence of other children at home, breast- or bottle-feeding, or hemoglobin concentration. Similarly, a study of 465 postpartum women also found that sleep problems predicted depression (Chaudron et al., 2001). In this sample, twenty-seven women became clinically depressed. At one month postpartum, four factors predicted depression at four months: trouble falling asleep, maternal age, depression during pregnancy, and thoughts of death and dying. In a population study of women at six to seven months postpartum, Brown and Lumley (2000) also found that tiredness was significantly related to depression.

In a sample of forty-one breastfeeding mothers (Wambach, 1998), fatigue moderately correlated with depression, perceived stress, and breastfeeding problem severity. These measures were taken at three days and three, six, and nine weeks postpartum. As predicted, fatigue was also correlated with depression at each time period. Older mothers and those whose babies had difficult temperaments also reported the highest levels of fatigue. Fatigue had no apparent impact on activities of daily living and maternal role activities.

Hypothyroidism

Sleep deprivation is the most obvious source of fatigue. But there are other causes. Another line of research examines the role of thyroid function in postpartum depression. Thyroxin is a hormone that regulates our metabolism. Low thyroid function can cause a wide range of depression-like symptoms including an inability to concentrate, tiredness, and forgetfulness. Low thyroid can also cause an intolerance to cold, persistently low body temperature, low blood pressure, weight gain, puffy face and eyes, constipation, and dry hair and skin.

Several studies found a connection between postpartum depression and postpartum hypothyroidism for some mothers. One study included 147 women, 22 of whom were diagnosed with major depression. Thyroid function was assessed by measuring levels of free thyroxine (fT4), triiodothyronine (fT3), and thyrotropin (TSH). At six to eight weeks postpartum, there was a higher incidence of depression in women with thyroid dysfunction (Harris et al., 1989). Three of the eight mothers who were diagnosed with postpartum thyroid dysfunction had major depression. The authors concluded that postpartum thyroid dysfunction often goes undetected because women attribute symptoms to postpartum fatigue.

An earlier study (Hayslip et al., 1988) had similar findings. The authors of this study followed fifty-one women for six months postpartum and noted substantial psychiatric morbidity in women who developed postpartum hypothyroidism. The symptoms they noted in particular included impaired concentration and memory and a subjective difficulty in performing work.

In a review of the literature on postpartum hypothyroidism, Weetman (1997) states that refractory depression is one indication for thyroid screening. He also noted that not every postpartum woman needs to be screened for hypothyroidism. However, women with insulin-dependent diabetes mellitus were three times more likely to develop postpartum hypothyroidism than nondiabetic women. Postpartum depression is also more common in women with thyroid antibodies, irrespective of biochemical thyroid dysfunction. Weetman recommended that women who develop postpartum thyroiditis should be screened for the next three to five years after birth, since approximately 25 percent of these women will develop hypothyroidism within five years. In another review, Pedersen (1999) also noted that lower range total and free thyroxine concentrations during late pregnancy are related to depression in the postpartum period.

A more recent study, however, has failed to find a link between postpartum depression and postpartum thyroid dysfunction (Lucas, Pizzaro, Granada, Salinas, & Santmarti, 2001). This study recruited 641 women during their thirty-sixth week of pregnancy and followed them through the first year postpartum ($N = 444$ at the twelve-month assessment). The authors found that fifty-six women (11 percent) developed postpartum thyroid disorder. None of these women were diagnosed with postpartum depression (using the Beck Depression Inventory). Their sample's rate of postpartum depression was abnormally low (1.7 percent), but they did find that women with a history of postpartum depression were significantly more likely to become depressed again.

Given the results of these studies, universal screening for hypothyroidism does not seem necessary. But it is a low-risk test and can be useful for mothers who are overly tired, or whose depression seems resistant to treatment.

Sleep Deprivation and Psychosis

Although psychosis is not the main focus of this book, it is important to mention here since sleep deprivation can have an impact on its development. Sleep deprivation has been related to delusional thinking and other psychotic symptoms in men and nonpostpartum women. Is it any surprise that it could have this same effect on women who have recently given birth? Personal accounts of postpartum psychosis (Skinner, 1991) and accounts given by women interviewed for this book who developed psychosis indicated that women who developed psychosis had been unable to sleep for two to three days before the onset of their illness. I consider inability to sleep a red-flag symptom that requires immediate medical attention. Charlotte describes her experience.

My second postpartum experience was a nightmare. I was exhausted. . . . I decided to wean my baby at two months because I was so exhausted and depressed. . . . I thought about suicide, institutionalization, and separation from my family constantly. . . . That postpartum psychosis exists was such a revelation to me because in April I had experienced a week of near-total insomnia. During these truly sleepless nights, I had no control over my thoughts, as if my brain had been put in a food processor. The first half of a thought would be rational and the second half would be totally unrelated, nonsensical.

The exact mechanism for the sleep deprivation-psychosis link is unclear at this time. Psychosis could be the result of biochemical changes resulting from lack of sleep. Or the lack of sleep may be due to an underlying condition, such as bipolar disorder. Surprisingly, the sleep deprivation-psychosis connection has not been studied with postpartum women. It has, however, been studied in other populations of patients, such as those with Parkinson's disease. Larsen and Tandberg (2001) noted that depression is a common risk factor for insomnia and poor sleep quality in patients with Parkinson's disease. The majority of problems of these patients could be traced to disordered REM sleep, and the symptoms ranged from vivid dreaming to psychosis.

In a study that sought to identify a biological marker for psychotic depression (Stefos et al., 1998), forty-four patients with nonpsychotic major depression were compared with forty-four patients with psychotic major depression. Sleep-related biological markers were significantly more common in the psychotic depressed patients. These included increased wakefulness, diminished REM latency, hypercortisolism, and blunted thyroid-stimulating hormone response to thyrotropin-releasing hormone stimulation. Shortened REM latency (when REM sleep predominates) was not influenced by severity but was related to psychosis along with the symptoms of depression.

The sleep-psychosis connection has also been described in case studies. One classic case study of sleep deprivation involved a New York disc jockey named Peter Tripp. In January 1959, Tripp endeavored to stay awake for 200 hours in a glass booth in Times Square as a fund-raiser for the March of Dimes. Below are excerpts from the government report on what happened to him.

> Almost from the first, the desire to sleep was so strong that Tripp was fighting to keep himself awake. After little more than 2 days and 2 nights, he began to have visual illusions; for example, he reported finding cobwebs in his shoes. By about 100 hours the simple daily tests that required only minimal mental agility and attention were a torture for him. He was having trouble remembering things, and his visual illusions were perturbing: he saw

the tweed suit of one of the scientists as a suit of fuzzy worms . . .
The daily tests were almost unendurable for Tripp and those
who were studying him. "He looked like a blind animal trying to
feel his way through a maze." A simple algebraic formula that
he had earlier solved with ease now required such superhuman
effort that Tripp broke down, frightened at his inability to solve
the problem, fighting to perform. Scientists saw the spectacle of
a suave New York radio entertainer trying vainly to find his way
through the alphabet.

By 170 hours the agony had become almost unbearable to
watch. At times Tripp was no longer sure he was himself, and
frequently tried to gain proof of his identity. Although he be-
haved as if he were awake, his brain wave patterns resembled
those of sleep. In his psychotic delusions he was convinced that
the doctors were in a conspiracy against him to send him to jail.
. . . At the end of the 200 sleepless hours, nightmare hallucina-
tion and reality had merged, and he felt he was the victim of a sa-
distic conspiracy among the doctors. (Luce, 1966, pp. 19-20)

Tripp recovered fairly quickly after he had about thirteen hours of
sleep, but he complained of depression for about three months after.
His experience had a number of similarities to those of the women
suffering from postpartum psychosis, including delusions, hallucinations, and paranoia. It is interesting too that this case study described
a man, who would not be subject to the same hormonal influences
common in postpartum or menstruating women, yet he manifested
symptoms similar to those of women suffering from postpartum psychosis. It is important to note that not everyone who is sleep deprived
develops symptoms of psychosis, but it could be a catalyst for women
who are already vulnerable. Judy, a labor and delivery nurse, describes how sleeplessness preceded her bout with postpartum psychosis. She was initially diagnosed with schizophrenia. Her diagnosis was later changed to bipolar disorder. She was hospitalized for
twenty-eight days.

In the months after her birth I often was easily overwhelmed. Fatigue did
not vanish. Fears of losing her, my boys, and/or [my husband] grasped me
frequently. . . . Exhaustion came, but I did not submit. After [my daughter] was
asleep, thoughts bombarded me for hours only to awake alert at 4 or 5 a.m.
. . . The week after the [childbirth education] seminar, sleeplessness continued. A whimper or sneeze from one of my children would jar me into a state

of alertness. Racing thoughts about the deficits of the maternity care system in the U.S. or my childhood bombarded my mind. I'd enter their room . . . hoping one of the three would be awake. Usually they weren't so I spent hours formulating and recording plans and ideas. . . . As the week progressed, I became less functional. We delayed leaving for a camping trip Thursday night since I was unable to accomplish packing. [My husband] received phone calls from relatives telling him of the strange content of the lengthy long-distance calls I'd placed. He forbade me to use the phone. I continued, though, because I sensed a great urgency of my thoughts.

Sleep Intervention

In an effort to improve the mental health of mothers, researchers have tried two different sleep interventions. In the first, Hiscock and Wake (2002) implemented a program aimed at improving infant sleep. In this intervention, parents were instructed in a "controlled crying" intervention, in which they were instructed to wait a longer and longer period before they responded to their infants. Depressed mothers in the intervention group were significantly less depressed two months later, and these mothers sustained their lower depression scores at four months.

Although these results look promising, researchers have raised some serious questions about the appropriateness of this technique (Mathews & Baker, 2002; Perl, 2002). For example, Perl (2002) compares this program to a "Nazi drill."

As a German, I am unhappy to find fairly undiluted ideas of militaristic Nazi infant care uncritically repeated by these Australian care providers. The Nazis understood very well the crucial effect of letting young babies cry on their future development and made this a central theme in their child care. As a scientist, I find it hard to believe that all of the results of mother-infant sleep research of the 1990s completely escaped the authors' notice.

We also need to balance the recommendations with the needs of the infant and the developing mother-infant relationship. Perhaps we may find a more humane solution, such as cosleeping, that allows both mothers and babies to sleep better.

From a methodological standpoint, the study design also has limitations. The mothers in the control group received only a sheet giving them instructions about infant sleep, while the intervention group received personalized instruction over three sessions. Perhaps it was the human contact, rather than the intervention, that made the difference for these mothers (Lipman, 2002).

Another sleep intervention has been used with postpartum mothers. In this case, sleep deprivation was used to treat mothers (Parry et al., 2000). Nine women with major depressive disorder in either pregnancy or within the first year postpartum were deprived of sleep in either the early part of the night or the late part of the night. Mood was assessed before and after the intervention, and after a night of recovery sleep. The study revealed that more patients responded to late-night sleep deprivation, and their response was better after a night of recovery sleep. The authors concluded that well-timed sleep deprivation may be a helpful alternative treatment when standard treatments fail or are not appropriate for a particular patient.

Summary

Fatigue and sleep deprivation can be important signs or even triggers for postpartum depression and psychosis. Whereas most new mothers are tired, those who seem exceptionally tired and unable to cope may be depressed. Sleeplessness not related to baby care can be a particularly ominous sign that requires close monitoring. Fatigue is only one of the important physiological influences in depression. The immune system may also have a role.

IMMUNE SYSTEM FUNCTION AND DEPRESSION

One intriguing theory of depression has to do with the immune system. In a review article, Marshall (1993) put forth a hypothesis that immune system function (allergies in particular) could be one pathway to depressive symptoms. Allergic reactions share some similarities with dysfunctions of the hypothalamic-pituitary-adrenal axis and have to do with the action of acetylcholine.

Cholinergic Pathways in Depression

According to Marshall (1993), high levels of stress alter the balance between the neurotransmitters acetylcholine and norepinephrine, resulting in too much acetylcholine. Prolonged stress no longer inhibits cholinergic activity, which leads to secretion of the stress hormone cortisol. Cortisol levels are often elevated in people who are depressed.

The imbalance of acetylcholine also has a significant impact on sleep. Acetylcholine receptors and norepinephrine cells control the cycle of alternation of REM and non-REM sleep. REM sleep occurs when cholinergic activity is greater. When norepinephrine predominates, cholinergic cells are inhibited and the REM sleep period ends. Depressed patients exhibit disturbances in sleep continuity, reduced sleep efficiency, reduced slow-wave sleep, increased REM activity and density, and shortened REM latency. All of these may be due to changes in the balance between acetylcholine and norepinephrine (Marshall, 1993). These changes in sleep could also relate to the fatigue and sleep deprivation described in the previous section.

Depression and Cytokine Activity

Miller (1998) has also noted that the immune system may play a role in the pathophysiology of depression. He was particularly concerned with the impact of the cytokines—chemical messengers of the white blood cells (such as interleukin-1, IL-1). When proinflammatory cytokines circulate in the system, they mediate sickness behavior in humans, including alterations in sleep. These cytokines also stimulate the release of cortisol.

Cytokines and Immune Markers in Postpartum Women

Physical stress can lead to an increase in cytokine production. Not surprisingly, cytokine levels are often elevated in women after giving birth. One study found that postpartum women are generally higher in the cytokines IL-6, IL-6R, and IL-IRA than before delivery (Maes, Lin, et al., 2000). Another study (Corwin, Bozoky, Pugh, & Johnston, 2003) found that interleukin-1β (IL-1β) was related to fatigue in postpartum women. Corwin et al. collected measures of fatigue and urinary excretion of IL-1β over four weeks postpartum. The authors found that IL-1β is elevated during the postpartum period and that this elevation has a significant, though delayed, relationship to postpartum fatigue. IL-1β may have an indirect link to postpartum depression through fatigue.

In a study of ninety-eight pregnant women three days before delivery, and at one and three days postpartum, Maes, Libbrecht, and colleagues (2001) found that serum prolyl endopetidase (PEP) activity in women with a past history of depression differed from that of those who had not been depressed. Postpartum women who had a previous episode of postpartum major depression had significantly lower levels of PEP than women who were not depressed. The same was not true for postpartum women who had a history of minor depression.

These studies on the immune system are preliminary but of interest. They give us one more way to understand depression in postpartum women. They also underscore the complexity and interrelationships between biological pathways and depression.

PAIN

Pain is another risk factor for postpartum mental disorders that can stem from both biological and psychosocial causes. Much of what we know about the pain-depression connection comes from the general chronic pain literature. Yet this literature has relevance to the needs of postpartum women. For example, in a study of 120 HIV-positive men and women, constant pain was positively correlated with depression (Lagana et al., 2002).

Colegrave, Holcombe, and Salmon (2001) compared four groups of women: those with treatment-resistant breast pain, those with newly diagnosed breast pain, those with newly diagnosed pain but not seeking treatment, and women who were pain-free with breast lumps. They found that women with any type of breast pain were significantly more anxious and depressed than pain-free women. In another study (Ozalp, Sarioglu, Tuncel, Aslan, & Kadiogullari, 2003), researchers found that when women were recovering from breast surgery, pain intensity, total analgesic consumption, and the dose/demand ratio were significantly related to preoperative anxiety and depression. In short, people who were depressed and anxious before surgery had higher levels of postoperative pain and analgesic requirements.

After childbirth, women may experience pain from a variety of sources: abdominal incisions, uterine contractions, swollen or engorged breasts, cracked nipples, episiotomies and/or perineal lacerations, back pains and headaches from spinal or epidural anesthesia, and muscle aches and pains. This pain, although transitory, can be severe and frightening.

One study (Thompson et al., 2002) found that postpartum pain is common. In this large sample of mothers at eight weeks postpartum, 53 percent reported backache, 37 percent reported bowel problems, 30 percent reported hemorrhoids, 22 percent reported perineal pain, and 15 percent reported mastitis (breast inflammation). Postpartum pain is often undermedicated, as a study on analgesia for women who had forceps deliveries found (Peter, Janssen, Grange, & Douglas, 2001).

Nipple pain, relatively common when breastfeeding is poorly managed, can lead to premature weaning, even in mothers committed to breastfeeding (Schwartz et al., 2002). It can also have a psychological impact on mothers (Amir, Dennerstein, Garland, Fisher, & Farish, 1996). In this study, forty-eight lactating women with nipple pain were compared with sixty-five lactating women without nipple pain. The women with pain were significantly more likely to be depressed; 38 percent of women in the pain group scored above the threshold for depression compared with 14 percent in the control group. Similarly, women in the pain group had significantly higher scores on all mood factors on the Profile of Mood States. These included tension, depression, fatigue, confusion, and vigor. Once the pain resolved, the scores on these scales dropped to normal levels.

In a study of 465 women, Chaudron and colleagues (2001) found that women who reported ten or more somatic complaints were nearly three times more likely to develop depression than women who reported nine or fewer symptoms. They also found a linear relationship between postpartum depression and an increasing number of physical or somatic complaints. Women in pain were more likely to be depressed and anxious.

In a study of 109 women hospitalized in a private mother-baby unit (Fisher, Feekery, Amir, & Sneddon, 2002), pain was also an issue. In this sample, 41 percent reported that their postpartum pain was inadequately controlled, and 41 percent described nipple pain that persisted longer than one week. Also, 29 percent had experienced at least one episode of mastitis. A high degree of postpartum pain was also associated with depression at eight months postpartum in another study of primiparous women (Rowe-Murray & Fisher, 2001).

Mothers with preexisting pain conditions may find that depression amplifies their postpartum pain. Data from a large epidemiological study indicated that depression can exacerbate the effects of medical illness and may be an independent source of suffering. The researchers concluded that depression is comparable to arthritis, diabetes, and hypertension, and that depression and chronic illness can interact and amplify the effects of the medical illness, including chronic pain syndromes (Gaynes, Burns, Tweed, & Erickson, 2002).

The Pain-Depression Link

Chronic pain and depression have significant overlap and may share a common etiology. An intriguing question is why this is so. Manning (2002) notes that pain and depression may share a common monoamine synaptic pathway in the central nervous system. The neurotransmitters serotonin and norepinephrine appear to be important in both. These substances are often low in depressed individuals, and both modulate pain sensitivity via the descending pain pathway. The involvement of both neurotransmitters could also explain why tricyclic antidepressants, or others that address both serotonin and norepinephrine, are often more effective in treating chronic pain than ones that address only serotonin levels (e.g., SSRIs).

Another possible link between pain and depression is the impact of pain on sleep. Sayar, Arikan, and Yontem (2002) compared forty patients with chronic pain to forty healthy control subjects on sleep quality, depression, and anxiety. As predicted, the chronic pain patients had significantly poorer sleep quality, more depression, and more anxiety. Pain intensity, anxiety, and depression correlated significantly with poorer sleep quality. However, in a multivariate analysis, depression was the only factor that was significantly correlated with sleep—explaining 34 percent of the variance.

In conclusion, pain can be a potent trigger to postpartum depression, but our understanding of why this is so is only in the beginning phases. This research does suggest that we need to treat postpartum pain aggressively and teach mothers some strategies for dealing with their own pain. Letting mothers know that it is time-limited can also be helpful.

HORMONAL INFLUENCES

The hormonal theory of postpartum depression is the oldest and best known—especially among the general public. At present, we know that women undergo substantial changes in hormone levels in the immediate postpartum period. The bone of contention, however, is whether these changes are related to depression. Past research has produced mixed results.

Reproductive Hormones

Estrogen, progesterone, and their metabolites are the most studied hormones in relation to postpartum depression. Depression is hypothesized as being most likely to occur if estrogen and progesterone levels are low. There is a large drop in the levels of these hormones immediately after birth. Hormonal research has proceeded along several lines: studying the day-5 peak, comparing the hormone levels of depressed and nondepressed women, and treating depressed women with hormones. A summary of these studies follows.

The Day-5 Peak

The day-5 peak refers to the time in the immediate postpartum period when women are tearful and irritable, have difficulty concentrating, and are sleepless. These changes are said to correspond to the dramatic drop in progesterone, estradiol, and cortisol, with the most dramatic change around the fourth or fifth day postpartum (Harris et al., 1994). Studies on the day-5 peak have had mixed results.

In a study of eighty-one women in the first three weeks after childbirth, Kendell, McGuire, Connor, and Cox (1981) found a day-5 peak for self-reported ratings of depression, tears, and lability. This peak occurred regardless of when women left the hospital, for primiparous and multiparous women, for breast- and bottle-feeding women, and for women who had cesarean or vaginal deliveries (Kendell, Mackenzie, West, McGuire, & Cox, 1984).

In a prospective study of 120 women, the maternity blues were associated with high antenatal progesterone the day before delivery, and lower levels of progesterone from the day of delivery to the day of peak blues. The same pattern was not observed for cortisol. Women who had cesarean sections were excluded from the study. The authors described their findings as a "weak but significant" association between progesterone and the blues. They concluded that progesterone levels immediately following delivery are responsible for maternal mood, and they recommended possible treatment of mothers with progesterone (Harris et al., 1994).

Although we tend to see this pattern after birth, some have also pointed out that a similar pattern follows surgery. If true, the postsurgical reaction suggests a mechanism other than shifts in reproductive hormones. Levy's (1987) study addressed this issue specifically. Levy compared emotional reactions of puerperal women ($N = 37$), women who had had major surgery ($N = 28$), and women who had minor surgery ($N = 22$). The surgeries were not reproductively related. Her results revealed a similar pattern of distress for the puerperal women and women who had had major surgery. In fact, dysphoria was greater following major surgery than after childbirth. Furthermore, crying and depression peaked in the same way in the postoperative women as it did in the puerperal women, with many postoperative patients commenting that the blues occurred suddenly and unexpectedly around the fourth postoperative day.

In summary, in spite of some evidence, are a number of factors argue against a wholly hormonal explanation for the day-5 peak (Chalmers & Chalmers, 1986). For example, not every mother experiences these emotions, which we would expect since all mothers experience hormonal shifts postpartum. Furthermore, in some cultures, the majority of women do not experience the day-5 peak, suggesting that a woman's environment can modify a biological process (Stern & Kruckman, 1983). In addition, fathers and women who adopt children often experience a day-5 peak and depression but do not experience hormonal adjustments.

Hormone Levels in Depressed and Nondepressed Women

Another approach has been to compare the hormone levels of depressed and nondepressed women. In perhaps one of the most carefully controlled and comprehensive studies to date, O'Hara, Schlechte, Lewis, and Varner (1991) drew blood and urine samples from approximately 173 women (number of participants varied slightly from assessment to assessment) at thirty-four, thirty-six, and thirty-eight weeks gestation, and at days 1, 2, 3, 4, 6, and 8 postpartum. The authors studied levels of estradiol, free estriol, progesterone, prolactin, total cortisol, and urinary free cortisol. The depressed subjects in their sample ($N = 18$) showed significantly lower levels of estradiol at thirty-six weeks gestation and at day 2 postpartum, but no other significant differences were found. Specifically, there were no significant differences in levels of free estriol, total estriol, progesterone, prolactin, total plasma cortisol, or urinary free cortisol between depressed and nondepressed subjects at any of the other assessment periods. Furthermore, there were no significant differences between depressed and nondepressed subjects for ratios of prolactin to estradiol or progesterone for any of the assessments. The authors concluded that they saw little evidence of a hormonal influence in postpartum depression. O'Hara came to a similar conclusion in his 1995 review of the literature:

> In spite of a large sample size and accurate estimations of hormone levels, there was *weak support* for the hormonal hypothesis. In fact, on at least two postpartum days, in direct contrast to our prediction, measures of free and total estriol levels were significantly *higher* in women experiencing the blues than in women not experiencing the blues. (p. 134, emphasis added)

Researchers continue to study this phenomenon. In a more recent study, the authors were able to induce a postpartum depression-like syndrome in the laboratory. Bloch and colleagues (2000) recruited two groups of eight women: women with previous postpartum depression, and women with no history of postpartum depression. They simulated the high hormone levels of pregnancy and then withdrew the steroids under double-blind conditions. During withdrawal, 62.5 percent of the women with a history of postpartum depression developed significant mood symptoms. None of the comparison women were affected. The authors concluded that their findings constituted direct support for the involvement of reproductive hormones in the development of postpartum depression in a subgroup of women. They noted that women with a history of postpartum depression may be differentially sensitive to changes in these hormone levels and may respond with negative mood states. These findings are interesting, but need to be reproduced in a larger sample.

Treatment for Postpartum Conditions Using Hormones

The final strategy for studying postpartum hormonal influences involves treating women at risk for postpartum depression with hormones. Dalton (1985) gave progesterone prophylactically to 100 women who had previous episodes of postpartum depression, and compared them with 221 women who had also had prior postpartum depression but did not receive progesterone. The recurrence rate in women who received progesterone was 10 percent, compared with 68 percent of those who received no progesterone. These findings are striking, but the study had a major limitation: it was not double-blinded. The women and their doctors knew they were being treated. The findings could be due to the placebo effect. Moreover, women in the nontreatment group received nothing. The human contact, rather than the progesterone, could have been responsible for the finding.

Another group of researchers (VanderMeer, Loendersloot, & Van-Loenen, 1984) did conduct a double-blind placebo-controlled trial comparing progesterone suppositories with a placebo in ten women suffering from postpartum depression. There was no significant difference between the effect of the progesterone and the placebo. Indeed, when comparing subjective effects, three of the women preferred the placebo.

More recently, Ahokas and colleagues (Ahokas, Aito, & Rimon, 2000; Ahokas, Kaukoranta, Wahlbeck, & Aito, 2001) have used 17β-estradiol to treat severe postpartum depression and postpartum psychosis. In the study of depression (Ahokas et al., 2001), twenty-three women with postpartum major depression were recruited from a psychiatric emergency unit. All were severely depressed and had low serum estradiol concentrations. Within a week of treatment with estradiol, the depressive symptoms had substantially diminished, and by the end of the second week, when estradiol levels were comparable to the follicular phase, the scores on the depression measure were comparable to clinical recovery. The study of psychosis was similar (Ahokas et al., 2000). Ten women with postpartum psychosis all had very low levels of serum estradiol. Within a week of sublingual 17β-estradiol, symptoms were significantly improved. By the second week, when levels were almost normal, the women were almost completely free of psychiatric symptoms.

These studies are promising, but they have limitations. First, the trials were open label, which means everyone was aware of being treated. Was it the estradiol or the placebo effect? These studies raise some other questions, such as what are the normal levels of estradiol for postpartum women? Presumably, almost every woman is low in estradiol postpartum. How is it that only some become depressed or psychotic? Is there a certain level where we start to see psychiatric symptoms? Why are some women more vulnerable to these changes?

Summary

Despite the popularity of the hormonal explanation for postpartum depression, it has only limited scientific support. Future studies may find that reproductive hormones are indirectly related to depression because of their influence on stress hormones, immune markers, or sleep quality. In the meantime, in my opinion, there is not sufficient evidence to support treatment of postpartum depression with reproductive hormones—especially given some of the risks associated with their use.

Prolactin

Another hormone that changes dramatically in the puerperium is prolactin. Prolactin is the hormone associated with the onset and maintenance of lactation, and sharply rises postpartum. Researchers have also examined its possible role in depression.

In one study (Abou-Saleh, Ghubash, Karim, Krymski, & Bhai, 1998), data were collected from twenty-three pregnant women, seventy postpartum women (at seven days postpartum), and thirty-eight nongravid controls. Postpartum women had significantly greater levels of cortisol, prolactin, thyroxine, and estrogen than the nongravid women. The women with postpartum depression had significantly lower plasma prolactin levels than those who were not depressed. Women who breastfed were significantly less depressed than those who did not. Also, women with previous episodes of depression had significantly lower prolactin and TSH levels than those who not been previously depressed.

In a review on the role of prolactin in depression, Nicholas, Dawkins, and Golden (1998) found that evidence on the role of prolactin in depression was inconsistent. But prolactin appears to have an indirect effect because it regulates the release of serotonin.

Prolactin, Depression, and Breastfeeding

Because prolactin is so strongly associated with lactation, researchers have also considered whether breastfeeding women are more or less vulnerable to postpartum depression. Mezzacappa and Katkin (2002) presented data from two studies which indicated that breastfeeding buffers mothers against negative mood. In the first study, they compared twenty-eight breastfeeding and twenty-seven bottle-feeding mothers on levels of perceived stress in the past month. As predicted, the breastfeeding mothers reported less stress, even after controlling for possible confounding variables. In the second study, twenty-eight mothers who were both breast- and bottle-feeding were compared immediately after breastfeeding, and after bottle-feeding. The authors were trying to account for some of the confounds typically found in breastfeeding research (such as preexisting differences in mothers who chose to breast- rather than bottle-feed). They found that the act of breastfeeding was associated with a decrease in negative mood, and bottle-feeding was found to be associated with a decrease in positive mood in the same women.

In a study of 790 women at eight to nine months postpartum, Astbury, Brown, Lumley, and Small (1994) found that women who did not breastfeed from birth, or who were not breastfeeding at three months postpartum, were significantly more likely to be depressed. This effect could be due to inadequate support in the hospital or after discharge.

Depression and Breastfeeding Cessation

Researchers have also examined the role of breastfeeding cessation in depression. But did cessation lead to depression, or did depression lead to cessation? In a study from Barbados, Galler, et al. (1999) found that depressive symptoms at seven weeks postpartum predicted a reduced preference for breastfeeding at their infants' current and later ages. In a study of fifty-one postpartum women with major depression, Misri, Sinclair, and Kuan (1997) found that 83 percent of the women reported that depression preceded the cessation of their breastfeeding. Only 17 percent reported that depression began after they stopped breastfeeding.

In a study from England (Bick, MacArthur, & Lancashire, 1998), 906 women were interviewed forty-five weeks after delivery. In this sample, 63 percent had breastfed, but 40 percent of them had stopped within three months. The predictors of early cessation included depression, return to work within three months, and regular child care from female relatives.

A sample from Pakistan yielded similar results (Taj & Sikander, 2003). In this sample were 100 women with breastfeeding-age children ranging from two months to two years. Of these women, 38 percent had stopped breastfeeding, and their score on the Urdu version of the Hospital Anxiety and Depression Scale (HADS) averaged 19.66, compared with 3.27 for the breastfeeding women. Of the women who had stopped breastfeeding, 36.8 percent reported that their depression had preceded cessation of breastfeeding. The authors concluded that maternal depression causes mothers to stop breastfeeding.

At this point, it appears that we have stronger evidence that depression precedes breastfeeding cessation than the other way around. Some evidence also shows that breastfeeding may be protective of maternal mood.

CHOLESTEROL

The final biological factor I describe is cholesterol. Cholesterol is the precursor to many hormones and appears to be related to depression as well. The data came to light in nonpostpartum studies of cholesterol-lowering drugs and increased risk of suicide (Brunner, Parhofer, Schwandt, & Bronisch, 2002). Preliminary findings suggest a link because of abnormalities in serotonin levels when cholesterol is low (Brunner et al., 2002). Although this link is not proven, it is a fascinating possibility that applies to postpartum women (Brown, 1996; Brunner et al., 2002).

Cholesterol levels rise dramatically during pregnancy—as much as 43 percent—and decline rapidly after birth (Troisi et al., 2002). The process by which cholesterol influences mood is hypothesized because of its role in the production, reuptake, or metabolism of neuro-

transmitters. Serotonin, in particular, has been related to low or lowered cholesterol levels (Troisi et al., 2002). Estrogen also lowers cholesterol levels (Luckas, Buckett, Aird, & Kingsland, 1997).

Two studies have found a link between lowered cholesterol levels
and postpartum depression. The first study included twenty primiparous women (Ploeckinger et al., 1996). It showed a significant
correlation between the decrease in cholesterol and an increase in depressive symptoms. This finding remained even after controlling for
level of progesterone. It was not the absolute level of cholesterol that
was related to depression. Rather, it was the relative change in the levels that correlated with depressive symptoms.

In the second study, Troisi et al. (2002) found a similar link between serum cholesterol and mood in postpartum women. The sample was forty-seven healthy primiparous women. They were interviewed late in their pregnancies and early in the postpartum period.
The authors found that lower postpartum total cholesterol levels were
related to anxiety, anger, hostility, and depression. Lower postpartum
levels of HDL cholesterol were associated with anxiety.

However, another study (Coutu, Dupuis, & D'Antono, 2001) did
not find a link between negative mood and cholesterol lowering. Indeed, in some cases, lowering cholesterol led to lower anxiety levels.
So although these studies raise some interesting possibilities, they do
not completely explain postpartum mood disturbances.

CONCLUSION

Research on the biological underpinnings of depression in general,
and postpartum depression in particular, has exploded since the first
edition of this book was released in 1992. In the original edition, I had
to draw from other literatures to make statements about the impact of
sleep deprivation, fatigue, and pain on postpartum women. Now,
many excellent studies show how these physiological phenomena affect the mental well-being of mothers.

Researchers to date have not established that puerperal hormonal
changes are related to postpartum depression. The research that did
find hormonal effects used small samples of women, and some of the
studies had serious methodological difficulties including lack of control groups and lack of double-blind design. These limitations were
highlighted earlier in this chapter.

The good news is that our models of the biological influences in depression have grown much more sophisticated, due in part to the massive increase in information in neuroscience. We are only in the early stages of understanding the complex interplay between sleep, the immune system, reproductive hormones, cholesterol, and neurotransmitters.

The information on the mood-protecting effects of breastfeeding is good news to those of us who work with breastfeeding mothers. However, this news must be tempered with the impact of fatigue and pain in breastfeeding mothers. These women are still vulnerable, and we should take every step to help them overcome barriers to successful breastfeeding if we are concerned about their emotional well-being.

Future research promises to bring us to an even better understanding of how physiological factors can shape mood. In the next chapter, I describe another major risk factor for postpartum depression—negative birth experiences.

Chapter 4

Negative Childbirth Experiences

> The birth of a child, especially a first child, represents a landmark event in the lives of all involved. For the mother particularly, childbirth exerts a profound physical, mental, emotional, and social effect. No other event involves pain, emotional stress, vulnerability, possible physical injury or death, permanent role change, and includes responsibility for a dependent, helpless human being. Moreover, it generally all takes place within a single day. It is not surprising that women tend to remember their first birth experiences vividly and with deep emotion. (Simkin, 1992, p. 64)

In her landmark study, Simkin (1991, 1992) described how women remember details of their deliveries years later. This study included twenty students in her childbirth education classes. She had them write about the births shortly after they occurred, followed up with them fifteen to twenty years later, and asked them to write about their experiences again. She found that women accurately remembered childbirth, and that these experiences had a lasting impact on how women felt about themselves as women and as mothers.

Quality of childbirth experience covers a whole range. Some women have wonderful experiences, while others have dreadful ones. In talking with mothers over the years, I have learned that negative childbirth experiences are more common than we would like to believe. Some mothers feel they have failed. Others feel betrayed by their partners, doctors, or their own bodies. Still others liken their childbirth experiences to a sexual assault.

How common are negative reactions? One national study has addressed this question (Genevie & Margolies, 1987). Subjects in this study were a nationally representative sample of 1,100 mothers, ages eighteen to eighty. Given the age range of the sample, a very wide range of experiences was covered. Still, 60 percent of the mothers described the births in predominantly positive terms. This group also included mothers who described their experiences in terms such as "tough, but worth it." However, 40 percent of mothers in this sample described their childbirths in predominantly negative terms. More concerning, 14 percent described them as "peak negative experiences"—one of the worst experiences of their lives. The depth of feeling was expressed in their narratives as well. Several of these women explained that childbirth had been so difficult that they had elected not to have any more children.

CHARACTERISTICS OF NEGATIVE CHILDBIRTH EXPERIENCES

Why do some women feel so badly about childbirth? Simkin (1991) describes how the subjective aspects of giving birth are often the most salient. Women who were most satisfied with their experiences felt that they had accomplished something important, that they were in control, and that the birth had significantly contributed to their sense of self-esteem and self-confidence. Women whose childbirths were not satisfying felt as if the experience had undermined their confidence, and they vividly recalled negative things that doctors or nurses said or did. In the next section, I highlight some of the subjective aspects of birth that have been related to negative reactions.

Sense of Control

Women's subjective sense of control is one of the most consistent predictors of positive feelings after childbirth. But this can be difficult to achieve in a hospital setting. Hospital environments tend to disempower patients (Rothman, 1982; Wertz & Wertz, 1989), and hospital deliveries, by their very nature, have many aspects that take away this sense of control. Women are stripped of their clothing and surrounded by strangers. Other people control their most basic functions, including when and what they eat and drink, whether they receive pain medication, and whether they can have a support person with them. They are likely to be subjected to a series of internal examinations and may be afraid to object for fear of being labeled a bad patient. Decisions about obstetric interventions are usually made without their input, and they often have little say about when they leave the hospital.

Simkin (1991) noted that for women, being in control included two specific elements. The first was self-control, which included feeling like they conducted themselves with discipline and dignity. The second aspect was feeling that they had control over what was happening to them. Some were still quite angry and disappointed by what doctors and nurses did to them. Indeed, Simkin noted, "the way a woman is treated by the professionals on whom she depends may largely determine how she feels about the experience for the rest of her life" (p. 210). This brings us to our next variable.

Supportive Environment

Another subjective variable is the mother's perceived level of care. In a study of 790 women at eight to nine months postpartum, Astbury and colleagues (1994) found that women were at increased risk of depression if they had a cesarean or assisted vaginal birth, were dissatisfied with their antenatal care, had an epidural or general anesthesia during delivery, or felt that pain control during labor was inadequate. The interpersonal aspects of care were also important. Women who described their caregivers as "fairly kind" or "unkind," or who had unwanted people present during the birth, were at increased risk for depression.

Another study (Rowe-Murray & Fisher, 2001) found that lack of support during labor increased the risk for depression. This study compared the experiences of 203 primiparous women. They had either vaginal delivery, assisted vaginal delivery, or cesarean section. The authors found three variables related to postpartum depression at eight months: a high degree of postpartum pain, a perceived lack of support during labor and childbirth, and a less than optimal first contact with their babies. These accounted for 35 percent of the variance in depression.

The following is a story I use frequently when I teach health care providers about negative childbirth experiences. It describes a delivery that was directly related to a mother's depression. I like to use this story because on paper this childbirth probably appears fine. But the mother's subjective experience of it was quite different. Elizabeth describes how the social environment of the hospital contributed to her psychic distress and physical pain.

I had twenty-five hours of labor. It was long and hard. I was in a city hospital. It was a dirty, unfriendly, and hostile environment. There was urine on the floor of the bathroom in the labor room. There were 100 babies born that day. I had to wait eight hours to get into a hospital room postdelivery. . . . There were ten to fifteen women in the postdelivery room waiting for a hospital room, all moaning, with our beds being bumped into each other by the nursing staff. I was taking Demerol for the pain. I had a major episiotomy. I was overwhelmed by it all and in a lot of pain. I couldn't urinate. They kept catheterizing me. My fifth catheterization was really painful. I had lots of swelling and anxiety because I couldn't urinate. My wedding ring was stuck on my finger from my swelling. The night nurse said she'd had patients that had body swelling due to not urinating and their organs had "exploded." Therefore, she catheterized me again. They left the catheter in for an hour and a half. There was lots of pain. My bladder was empty but they wouldn't believe me. I went to sleep and woke up in a panic attack. I couldn't breathe and I couldn't understand what had happened.

In Elizabeth's story, we see themes of helplessness, pain, and dissociation. This experience was still vivid when she described it to me, even though several years had elapsed since it occurred, and she had had a subsequent positive childbirth after this experience. It also occurred in a well-known hospital, where the medical care is purported to be top-notch.

Prior Characteristics of the Mother

The mother's previous experiences may also influence how she felt about the birth and may be related to developing postpartum depression. The characteristics of particular interest are prior traumatic events or prior episodes of depression. In a study from Finland (Saisto, Salmela-Aro, Nurmi, & Halmesmaki, 2001), the authors examined the relationship between disappointment with delivery and personality characteristics, socioeconomic status, prior depression, and fear of labor. They found that pain in labor and emergency cesarean sections were the strongest predictors of disappointment with delivery. Personality traits such as anxiety and neuroticism, and depression during pregnancy were the strongest predictors of postpartum depression. Women who had been depressed during their pregnancies were significantly more likely to be disappointed with their deliveries, and to develop postpartum depression.

Prior depression was also related to intensity of labor pain and perceived health. In an American study of seventy women (Dannenbring, Stevens, & House, 1997), depression, duration of labor, and the expectation that they would not need medications during labor predicted affective pain. Physician-predicted complications, induced labor, and the motivation to not use medications predicted pain intensity (McKee, Cunningham, Jankowski, & Zayas, 2001).

Obstetric complications during pregnancy also predicted depression in a French study of 441 pregnant women; postpartum depression was also related to obstetric complications. There was no relationship between depression, labor and delivery, and neonatal complications (Verdoux, Sutter, Glatigny-Dallay, & Minisini, 2002). In contrast, a study from Australia found no relation between obstetric complications and postpartum depression. But it did find a relationship between postpartum depression and psychosocial risk factors, including demographic characteristics, personality characteristics, psychiatric history, and current life stressors (Johnstone, Boyce, Hickey, Morris-Yates, & Harris, 2001).

Depression in late pregnancy also predicted obstetric and neonatal complications (Chung, Lau, Yip, Chiu, & Lee, 2001). In a prospective study of 959 women in Hong Kong, depression in the third trimester was associated with increased use of epidural anesthesia, higher rates of cesarean sections and instrumental vaginal deliveries, and infant admissions to neonatal intensive care units (NICUs). These effects were still present even after the authors controlled for pregnancy complications.

Prior trauma can also lead to subsequent pregnancy complications. In a study of 455 women with PTSD, and 638 comparison women, Seng and colleagues (2001) found that PTSD increased the risk of complications during pregnancy. The women with PTSD had significantly higher odds ratios for ectopic pregnancy, spontaneous abortion, hyperemesis, preterm contractions, and excessive fetal growth. They found no relationship between PTSD and labor variables.

All of this discussion focuses on childbirth experiences in general. It is now time to turn our discussion to a form of delivery that has been the focus of the majority of research on negative childbirth experiences: cesarean sections.

Cesarean Sections: Are They Always Negative?

For more than twenty years, there has been concern about the high rate of cesarean sections in industrialized nations. In 1985, the World Health Organization stated that 15 percent was the highest acceptable limit for national cesarean rates. They based this number on findings from countries with the world's lowest rates of perinatal mortality (World Health Organization, cited in Belizan, Althabe, Barros, & Alexander, 1999).

Many developed countries are above the recommended rate of cesarean sections. Belizan and colleagues (1999) calculated rates of cesarean sections for all Latin American countries (except Nicaragua, whose rates were unavailable). They found that twelve of the nineteen countries had rates ranging from 16.8 percent to 40 percent. Cesarean sections were more common in private versus public hospitals and were directly related to gross national product (i.e., were more common in wealthy countries).

There is not enough space here to debate the subject of whether cesareans are usually justified. I am concerned, however, about the psychological impact of this procedure. The dominant paradigm for studying the impact of childbirth on women's emotional health has used cesarean sections as the prototype of the negative experience, while vaginal childbirth is more commonly the positive one. As I have described, the issue is more complex than this simple distinction. But some studies have consistent findings about the impact of cesareans on women. These studies are described next.

In a prospective study of 272 Australian women, Fisher, Astbury, and Smith (1997) assessed the psychological outcomes of various types of birth. They found that the total number of obstetric interventions made little difference. But there were significant differences based on type of delivery. Women who had cesareans were significantly more likely to have negative moods and low self-esteem, whereas women who had spontaneous vaginal deliveries had the most positive moods. Women with assisted vaginal deliveries were somewhere between the two groups.

Fisher et al. (1997) noted several factors that were less than positive in cesarean births. Women who had cesareans were significantly less likely to have their partners present, to see their babies in the first five minutes after birth, or to hold them after delivery. Indeed, 31 percent did not get to hold their babies within the first eight hours after birth. These infants were not more likely to be admitted to the NICU, suggesting that separation of mothers and babies following cesarean sections was routine. Moreover, women who had cesareans were significantly more likely to require narcotic pain medication and to develop postpartum physical complications.

Personal control also varied by type of delivery in this study (Fisher et al., 1997): 56 percent of women who had unassisted vaginal deliveries felt that they had personal control over their deliveries, compared with 19 percent of the women who had cesarean births. There was no significant difference in the reactions of those who had emergency versus planned cesarean births. The authors concluded that operative childbirth carries "significant psychological risks rendering those who experience these procedures vulnerable to a grief reaction or to posttraumatic distress and depression" (p. 728). They felt that the prospective design allowed them to draw causal inferences and that the reactions of the women could not be attributed to preexisting symptoms.

In an Australian study of women admitted to a private mother-baby unit for psychiatric care, 53 percent had had operative deliveries (Fisher, Feekery, Amir, & Sneddon, 2002). In this sample, approximately half of the mothers indicated that childbirth was worse than they expected it to be, and that they were disappointed with their childbirth experiences (Fisher, Feekery, & Rowe-Murray, 2002). The percentage of mothers who were disappointed was 36 percent for the whole sample, but it varied by type of birth (66 percent for cesarean birth, 45 percent for assisted vaginal, and 20 percent for unassisted vaginal). Moreover, 52 percent reported that their postpartum obstetric care was not adequate (Fisher, Feekery, Amir, & Sneddon, 2002). Many of these mothers had had problems conceiving and/or difficult pregnancies: 6.5 percent had conceived through in vitro conception, 25 percent had invasive prenatal testing, and 26 percent had an antenatal admission.

Durik, Hyde, and Clark (2000) had contrasting findings. They compared women who had vaginal deliveries ($N = 74$), women who had planned cesareans ($N = 37$), and women who had unplanned cesareans ($N = 56$). The women were assessed at one, four, and twelve months postpartum. As predicted, women with unplanned cesareans appraised their deliveries more negatively than women with planned cesareans or vaginal deliveries at one and four months. But there were no differences by delivery type for postpartum depression or self-esteem.

Another large study ($N = 1,596$) of planned cesarean sections versus vaginal deliveries for breech presentation had similar findings. The authors found no significant difference in rates of postpartum depression between the two groups (Hannah et al., 2002). Both groups had a rate of approximately 10 percent. Breastfeeding rates were also high in both groups and not significantly different. Also, 78 percent of women found it easy or very easy to care for their infants, and approximately 82 percent of the total sample found adjusting to motherhood easy or very easy.

Some differences were found in how women perceived their experiences and what they liked or disliked about them. For example, women in the planned cesarean birth group liked being able to schedule their delivery, that their experience was not painful, and that they felt reassured about the health of their babies. Women in the planned vaginal group indicated that they liked that the births were natural, that they were able to actively participate in the births, and that recovery from childbirth was not difficult. Both groups felt reassured about their own health (Hannah et al., 2002).

In summary, the results of these studies indicate that cesarean births can cause negative reactions for women who experience them. Women who received ample support following their cesareans, and who felt they had input in the decision-making process, however, were significantly less likely to have negative reactions. These variations in response also indicate that it is not the procedure of cesarean delivery per se that causes negative reactions. Therefore, cesarean sections do not have to be bad if women are provided with support and reassurance and are involved in decisions that concern them.

NEGATIVE VERSUS TRAUMATIC CHILDBIRTH

In the previous sections, I described some of the factors that led to women having negative childbirth experiences. Many of these experiences can result in depression, without necessarily producing psychological trauma. However, giving birth can also produce traumatic stress reactions, and can lead to an additional diagnosis of PTSD. Even women who do not meet full criteria for PTSD may have some trauma symptoms, which can be troublesome. PTSD is not restricted to women who have cesareans; women who have vaginal deliveries can be traumatized too.

Diagnostic Criteria for PTSD

According to DSM-IV-TR criteria (American Psychiatric Association, 2000), a traumatic event is one in which the person felt that death or serious injury was possible for themselves or a loved one, and the person responded with fear, helplessness, or horror. In addition, symptoms must occur in each of these clusters:

1. *intrusion:* frequent reexperiencing of the event via nightmares or intrusive thoughts;
2. *avoidance:* numbing or lack of responsiveness to or avoidance of current events that remind patients of their trauma; and
3. *hyperarousal:* persistent symptoms of increased arousal, including jumpiness, sleep disturbances, or poor concentration. (Reprinted with permission from the *Diagnostic and Statistical Manual of Mental Disorders,* Fourth Edition, Text Revision (Copyright 2000). American Psychiatric Association, pp. 467-468.)

PTSD is acute if the symptoms have been present for less than three months and chronic if the symptoms have been present for three months or more. The onset of PTSD is considered "delayed" if it occurs six months or more after the initial stressor.

Childbirth As a Traumatizing Experience

Two studies have shown that some women develop PTSD after giving birth. In the first study, 289 women were followed prospectively. They were assessed at thirty-six weeks during pregnancy, and at six weeks and six months postpartum. Women with preexisting PTSD or depression were not included in the analyses. The authors found that at six weeks, 2.8 percent of women met full criteria for PTSD. At six months postpartum, 1.5 percent still met criteria, and had developed chronic PTSD (Ayers & Pickering, 2001).

In another study, 264 women with unassisted vaginal childbirth were assessed at seventy-two hours and six weeks postpartum (Czarnocka & Slade, 2000). Of these women, 3 percent met full criteria for PTSD, and had clinically significant levels of intrusive thoughts, avoidance, and hyperarousal. Furthermore, 24 percent had at least one symptom. The factors that predicted traumatic stress symptoms were similar to those that predicted depression. They included a low level of partner or staff support and low perceived control during labor.

The percentage of women who met full criteria for PTSD may at first seem small. But you should take some factors into account when considering these results. First, the authors of the first study (Ayers & Pickering, 2001) excluded all women with previous episodes of PTSD or depression—the very women most vulnerable to subsequent PTSD. If these women were included, the percentage would probably double. Second, in the weeks following the September 11, 2001, terrorist attacks on New York City, the rate of PTSD in Manhattan was 7.5 percent. People who suffered from previous episodes of depression and PTSD were not excluded from this estimate (Galea et al., 2003). This percentage is more than double the percentages in the previously cited birth studies. But it refers to the worst slaughter on American soil in more than a century. Birth, in contrast, is supposed to be a happy event. The fact that any women meet full criteria for PTSD should alert us that something is seriously amiss. The fact that 24 percent had some symptoms is quite concerning. As a culture, we probably need to rethink how we handle women in labor—especially those who are already vulnerable because of prior traumatic events.

A Model for a Trauma-Producing Experience

A model I have found helpful in understanding childbirth is Figley's (1986) conceptualization of characteristics of a trauma-producing event. According to Figley, events are troubling to the extent that they are sudden, dangerous, and overwhelming. These three characteristics have a great deal of relevance to birth, and can help you understand why a particular mother might be bothered by her experience. An event is sudden when it strikes without time to prepare, devise an escape plan, or prevent it. This certainly occurs when women are in the hospital and in labor; change can happen in seconds, and there may be little time to react.

Danger is the second element. Many women perceive that labor is life-threatening for themselves or their babies (Figley, 1986). In terms of PTSD, it is the mother's perception that matters, not whether her perceptions are medically "true." The situation is similar to that of a crime victim who believes that she will be killed—even if the criminal has no intention of killing her. What she believes is much more relevant to her subsequent reaction than the actual facts associated with the event.

The final element is the extent to which the situation is overwhelming. Some women describe being swept away by their childbirth experiences and the hospital routines. Being overwhelmed leads to a sense of temporary helplessness and being out of control. They are overwhelmed by what is happening and cut off from important information. The same can be true for their partners. Sally's emergency cesarean had all three aspects that are likely to put women at risk for traumatic stress reactions. Her baby was born within fifteen minutes of when the cord prolapsed after she had been in labor for twenty-three hours. Her delivery was by cesarean section under general anesthesia:

They had me on the bed, rear end in the air. My head was down between the headboard and the mattress. The nurse had to hold the baby off the cord. All I kept hearing was "OB emergency, OB emergency" over the loudspeaker, while the nurse kept saying in my ear that the baby would be fine. Everything happened so quickly; I didn't have time to react.

Risk Factors for a Trauma-Producing Birth

Women can come to childbirth with issues and past experiences that make them vulnerable to PTSD. These vulnerabilities are similar to those that lead to depression after a birth: prior depression, prior PTSD, previous high-risk pregnancy, and previous childbearing loss.

Prior Trauma

Prior trauma can make people more vulnerable to a current stressor. In a qualitative study of women who had been sexually abused as children, Rhoades and Hutchinson (1994) found that labor activated memories of past abuse. Some of the medical procedures, such as use of intravenous lines or fetal monitors, made them feel tied down or restrained, as they had been during assault. Similarly, Reynolds (1997) describes how some of the commands during labor, such as "open your legs," "cooperate," or "be a good girl" can remind women of their abuse experiences.

The notion that prior trauma creates vulnerability to subsequent events has support from the general trauma literature. In a representative sample of men and women in southeast Michigan ($N = 2,181$), Breslau, Chilcoat, Kessler, and Davis (1999) found that a history of trauma was associated with a greater risk of PTSD from the index event. Those who had experienced multiple traumas were at greater risk than those who had experienced a single trauma. Prior assaultive trauma, either in childhood or later on, was particularly damaging. In citing other studies, Breslau et al. also described how previous major depression can also predispose people to PTSD.

Prior trauma may also influence how pregnancy is experienced and how many symptoms mothers develop. For example, a case-control study of eighty-two women with low-birth-weight infants, and ninety-one women with normal-weight babies, assessed women for a history of child sexual abuse. The sexually abused women were not more likely to have a low-birth-weight baby. However, they were more likely to smoke during pregnancy. They also tended to have more health complaints during pregnancy and used more antenatal health care services, but they did not have more obstetric complications (Grimstad & Schei, 1999). Symptoms during pregnancy that were more common among abuse survivors included heartburn and regurgitation, feeling tired or faint, uterine contractions, back pain, and numbness or tingling of fingers and hands.

Pregnancy Loss and High-Risk Pregnancy

Traumatic experiences can also include a history of childbearing loss. Women may have had previous ectopic pregnancies, stillbirths, or miscarriages. This may make them feel that they cannot deliver their babies. Sometimes women who have had previous negative childbirth experiences can only remember their deliveries with sadness, anger, pain, or fear. A highly detailed birth plan may also indicate a trauma history during which a woman felt completely out of control in a previous situation. Her detailed plan may be an attempt to regain some of this lost control.

Not surprisingly, prior infant loss can increase the risk of depression and PTSD. Janssen, Cuisinier, Hoogduin, and de Graauw (1996) compared 227 women whose babies had died with 213 who gave birth to live babies. Six months later, women whose babies had died showed greater depression, anxiety, and somatization than women who had given birth to live babies. At one year, the mental health symptoms had subsided, and the women who lost babies appeared comparable to those who had not lost babies. However, the authors noted that pregnancy loss is a stressful life event that can lead to a marked deterioration in a woman's mental state, particularly in the first six months.

Having a prior stillbirth can also lead to depression and anxiety in a subsequent pregnancy (Hughes, Turton, & Evans, 1999). This study compared women who had a previous stillbirth with a group of matched controls ($N = 82$). Women who had a stillbirth had more depression and anxiety in their third trimesters, and more depression postpartum. The results were strongest for women who were most recently bereaved. Not surprisingly, depression during pregnancy was highly predictive of postpartum depression. In the year following delivery, 8 percent of the control group and 19 percent of the bereaved women scored high for depression.

Mothers who come into childbirth having had these types of prior experiences are going to be very vulnerable to even routine care. If difficulties occur in their deliveries, the women may develop full-blown PTSD.

Trauma-Producing Births: One Woman's Story

Following are the stories of Kathy's two deliveries. Each one was difficult for different reasons. According to Reynolds (1997), two aspects of labor make it potentially traumatizing: extreme pain and loss of control. These stories have both of these elements. Kathy experienced fear of dying, overwhelming pain, and experiences that overpowered her. She also experienced a replaying of events afterward.

When Peter was born, the birth itself was pain free. He was small, especially his head and shoulders, and it truly didn't hurt at all. I kept insisting I wasn't really in labor up until two minutes before he was born, when the doctor told me to lay down, shut up, and push! But afterward—he was born at 9:30—they told us he had Down syndrome at noon, and by 4 p.m., I was hemorrhaging so badly that I came within two minutes of death. I had to have an emergency D&C with no anesthesia (talk about PAIN!!) and a big blood transfusion.

That night, they told us Peter needed immediate surgery and had to go to a hospital in another city. A very traumatic day, to say the least. And then they sent me home the next day with no mention at all that I might want to talk to somebody about any of this—the Down syndrome, the near-death experience, nothing. I can still call up those memories with crystal clarity. And whenever we hear about another couple, I have to reprocess those feelings. Interestingly, most of them relate to the hemorrhaging and D&C, not to the Down syndrome "news." They're all tied up together. Maybe it's good to remind myself every so often of how precious life is.

My third birth was excruciatingly painful—the baby was nine pounds, three ounces, with severe shoulder dystocia—his head was delivered twenty minutes before his shoulders. I had some Stadol in the IV line right before transition, but that's all the pain relief I had. I thought I was going to die, and lost all perspective on the fact that I was having a baby. I just tried to live through each contraction. Of course, I was flat on my back, with my feet up in stirrups, and watching the fetal monitor as I charted each contraction—I think those things should be outlawed! I know now that if I had been squatting, or on my hands and knees, I probably could have gotten him out much easier. I'm the one who has the giant shoulders and incredibly long arms, so I can't blame anyone else for my two babies with broad shoulders (Miranda, the first, also took several extra pushes to get her shoulders out, but she was "only" eight pounds, one ounce).

That night, after Alex was born (at nine in the morning), I could not sleep at all because every time I tried to go to sleep, my brain would start rerunning the tape of labor, and I would feel the pain and the fright and the fears of dying all over again. I stayed up all that night and the next day, and didn't sleep until I was home in my own bed.

In Kathy's stories, we see some classic symptoms of a post-traumatic stress response: the fear of dying, the sleeplessness, and the reexperiencing of labor, both immediately afterward and when someone had a similar experience. She did eventually come to a place of peace over her experiences, but the memories of those two episodes of labor have remained vivid.

Difficult Births and Breastfeeding

The two most common sequelae of negative childbirth experiences are depression and PTSD. One other consequence often is not considered but could have ramifications for both mother and baby. A difficult birth can influence a mother's ability to breastfeed. Two studies have specifically examined this issue.

The first study (Grajeda & Perez-Escamilla, 2002) used a sample of 136 urban women from Guatemala. Grajeda and Perez-Escamilla measured the women's cortisol levels before and after giving birth. They found that primiparous women had higher cortisol levels overall, and cortisol levels were substantially elevated after birth. For women with the higher levels of cortisol, lactation onset was delayed by several days.

The second study (Rowe-Murray & Fisher, 2002) was prospective and included 203 primiparous women. These women were interviewed at two days postpartum and completed a survey at eight months postpartum. The authors found that women who had cesarean sections often waited several hours to initiate breast-feeding compared with women who delivered vaginally, either with or without assistance. The one hospital in the study that had World Health Organization designation as "baby-friendly" had a shorter delay—but it was still a delay. On a positive note, the delay in initiation of lactation was not related to continuation of breastfeeding at eight months.

THE EFFICACY OF DEBRIEFING

In this section, I describe one intervention that has received some attention with regard to negative birth experiences (other trauma-focused treatments are described in Chapters 10 and 11). For women who have had emotionally difficult childbirth, debriefing has been tried. During debriefing, a midwife talks to women and allows them to ask questions and discuss any feelings of sadness, guilt, anger, or confusion. The results have been mixed as to whether debriefing is helpful to mothers.

In one randomized trial, mothers in England were randomly assigned to a debriefing ($N = 56$) or standard care ($N = 58$) condition (Lavender & Walkinshaw, 1998). Midwives provided debriefing that included listening, support, counseling, understanding, and explanation of treatment. At three weeks postpartum, those who received the intervention were significantly less likely to be anxious or depressed.

In contrast, an Australian study of 917 women who had had either cesarean section or vaginal delivery using forceps or vacuum extraction found that a higher percentage of debriefed women were depressed and in poorer health at six months postpartum than women assigned to standard care. These differences between the groups were not significant, however. Indeed, the overall percentages of depressed women were small (17 percent versus 14 percent for debriefed versus standard care respectively; Small, Lumley, Donohue, Potter, & Waldenstrom, 2000). Interestingly, these results occurred even though mothers reported that the intervention had been helpful to them. A higher percentage also reported that depression had been a problem for them since the delivery (28 percent versus 22 percent). The authors concluded that debriefing was ineffective and could even be harmful.

In discussing this study, Boyce and Condon (2001) noted some methodological points that temper these findings. First, they noted that debriefing is for the prevention of PTSD, not depression. Thus, it is not surprising that this intervention did not have an impact. They also noted that women who had had elective versus emergency procedures were grouped together, and that may have obscured the findings. Finally, they questioned the usefulness of having a midwife debrief who had not been present at the birth. They wondered how she could answer women's questions when she had not been there. They also pointed out that even though this particular intervention was not effective, women need the opportunity to discuss their experiences.

A review (Gamble, Creedy, Webster, & Moyle, 2002) of midwife-led debriefing found insufficient evidence as to the effectiveness of debriefing. The methodological issues Gamble et al. raised included a lack of a standardized debriefing intervention, a lack of comprehensive outcome variables including the noninclusion of trauma symptoms, and lack of inclusion of the woman's partner in the debriefing. The authors concluded that a single-session intervention would probably be insufficient to deal with the problem. But they acknowledged that talking to someone about the experience may have had some benefit. On the other hand, women who had been most deeply traumatized by childbirth may have been so numb from the experience, or may have desired so strongly to just get back to normal, that any intervention immediately after the experience would have been pointless.

Astbury et al. (1994) also explained how women might reevaluate childbirth after the initial danger has passed and the crisis of the first few months has resolved. Particularly in a birth with a large amount of intervention, the initial reaction may simply be happiness that they survived the experience. Only later may they allow themselves to question some of what was done in the hospital. This could create a delayed response, so that in subsequent months the birth is viewed more negatively.

Simkin (1992) echoes this possible explanation. In exploring the nature of memory changes over a length of time, she noted that a halo often occurs shortly after giving birth, women gloss over negative parts of their experiences in their initial euphoria. With time, the halo fades and aspects of childbirth are looked at more realistically. Because of this delay, caregivers are usually blithely unaware of the consequences of their actions for the women they serve. Many providers do not realize that women are often quite upset by their actions and that these negative feelings can last for years.

CONCLUSION

Women who have had traumatic or difficult childbirth experiences must acknowledge their trauma if they are ever to move past it. Trying to "just forget it" is not an effective strategy, and trauma that is not acknowledged and dealt with will manifest itself in a variety of destructive and negative behaviors. Women who have not processed their experience may manifest symptoms such as depression, blunted affect and inability to empathize with others (including their infants), helplessness, self-destructive behaviors, somatic complaints, sexual dysfunctions, marital difficulties, anger, and hostility. They may also become pregnant again before they are physically and emotionally ready in order to do things differently "this time." Working through trauma is difficult, but it is the only route to healing.

As a result of working through trauma, a woman acknowledges and gives herself permission to feel pain and anger following her experience. She may need a period of time to grieve over her experience. As trauma and grief are reclaimed, she can give meaning to the events and move forward. She may even come to value her experience and try to do something to help other people. This is what one article (Wilson & Zigelbaum, 1986) described as the healthiest form of coping with psychological trauma.

In conclusion, the research literature on recovery from traumatic events contains a message of hope: people can and do recover from psychological trauma. The most important components of any intervention focus on helping women acknowledge and accept their experiences, and on helping them regain a sense of efficacy.

An article written specifically for mothers is available on my Web site: <www.GraniteScientific.com>. It is titled "Making Peace with Your Birth Experience."

Chapter 5

Infant Characteristics
and Depression in Their Mothers

Developmental psychologists once believed that mothers influenced their babies, but babies did not influence their mothers. Then researchers discovered what now seems glaringly obvious: babies bring quite a lot to the interaction, and could indeed be a major influence on their mothers' emotional state. Two infant characteristics in particular influence mothers: infant temperament and infant health status.

INFANT TEMPERAMENT

Babies bring their own personalities to their relationships with their mothers. Babies' personalities include how much they cry, how shy they are, how distractible, irritable, soothable, and active. Infant personality is more commonly known as infant temperament. Broadly defined, temperament is a behavioral style and characteristic way of responding to people and the environment (Campos, Bartlett, Lamb, Goldsmith, & Stenberg, 1983).

The most commonly cited work on infant temperament is that of Chess and Thomas (1977; Thomas & Chess, 1987). Based on their research, Chess and Thomas described infant temperament as falling into three basic types: easy, difficult, and slow to warm up. In their longitudinal study, Chess and Thomas (1977) classified 40 percent of the children as easy, 10 percent as difficult, and 15 percent as slow to warm up. The remaining 35 percent were somewhere between these three categories. Thomas and Chess (1987) conceptualized temperament as a stable characteristic of newborns that is later shaped and modified by the child's experiences.

The child with a difficult temperament is central to our study of the infant's impact on postpartum depression. Difficult infants have strong emotional reactions; cry for long periods of time; are hard to comfort; are slow to accept new people, foods, or routines; and are less easy to predict or regulate in their eating, sleeping, or elimination schedules. Mothers might describe these babies as "colicky" (Canivet, Jakobsson, & Hagander, 2002; Cutrona & Troutman, 1986). In one diary study of newborns (Canivet et al., 2002), the rate of colic was 9.4 percent, similar to the percentage of babies identified as "difficult" by Chess and Thomas (1977). Babies with difficult temperaments can be challenging to care for. They are often unadaptable and irritable and can make mothers' efforts to soothe them seem ineffective. Mothers may conclude that they themselves are not effective or competent (Beck, 1996a) and begin to resent their babies. They are often afraid to share their feelings with others, as this mother describes:

My first baby screamed from the day he was born. He screamed all the time, even in the hospital. He reacted oddly to all kinds of different things. The pediatrician said he was a "difficult" child. Even now, he has to have things always the same. . . . When I went back for a checkup at two weeks, a nurse asked me how the baby was. She said, "Aren't they wonderful?" I didn't know what to say. I thought he was the pits.

Not surprisingly, mothers of babies with difficult temperaments are more vulnerable to depression. In a study of forty-three mothers of thirteen-month-olds (Levitt, Weber, & Clark, 1986), mothers with difficult infants were more likely to be depressed and report less satisfactory relationships with their husbands than were mothers of easy infants. Bond, Prager, Tiggemann, and Tao (2001) found similar results. In their study of 116 mothers of colicky babies, they found high levels of psychological distress and anxiety. The mothers reported low self-efficacy, low levels of attachment to the baby, and less satisfaction with their lives since having their babies. Social support did not ameliorate the effects. Beck (1996a) conducted a meta-analysis of seventeen studies on infant temperament and postpartum depression. She found a moderate effect size for the relationship between a difficult infant temperament and depression in mothers (ranging from .31 to .36 for weighted and unweighted, respectively).

Cutrona and Troutman (1986) causally linked infant temperament to postpartum depression. They assessed fifty-five married women during pregnancy and at three months postpartum. The authors found that caring for a difficult infant gradually erodes a mother's feelings of competence as a parent and her overall sense of well-being. When a direct link between infant temperament and maternal depression was examined statistically, infant difficulty alone accounted for 30 percent of the variance in depression. Prolonged exposure to such infants may make their mothers feel ambivalent toward them, often resulting in guilt and self-hatred. When mothers feel this way, they often withdraw or can even become abusive. A temperamentally difficult infant may disrupt several aspects, as Barbara describes:

When the baby started throwing up, I felt terrible. I wouldn't go anyplace with her because I didn't want people to see her screaming. I wanted to be the perfect mother. . . . My mother-in-law said, "You've got to relax. She's picking up on your cues." . . . The baby had a difficult temperament. Even now, she's very stubborn and strong-willed. The control issue is big for me. I'm a perfectionist and always have been. I don't want the baby to experiment with food, even though I know it's normal. I don't want her to do it. . . . I wanted this baby so bad. When she came, I hated her. I thought of throwing her out the window. I just wanted her to die. I spanked her when she was three or four weeks old, and I'm still dealing with the guilt of it. . . . I'd yell at her, right in her face: "I hate you. I wish you would die."

In another study, women at high risk for postpartum depression were compared with a sample of women at low risk. Their infants were assessed in the neonatal period using the Neonatal Behavioral Assessment Scale. Babies' high irritability and poor motor skills strongly predicted maternal depression at eight weeks postpartum and poor infant behavior in face-to-face interactions (Murray, Stanley, Hooper, & King, 1996). These findings were true even after controlling for maternal mood in the neonatal period and for maternal perceptions of infant temperament.

Infant Crying

Infant crying is the most salient behavior in babies with difficult temperaments. Crying can be very difficult for new parents to cope with and is one of the most common reasons for pediatric visits in the first three months. Colic is usually diagnosed using the Wessel criteria: crying or fussing that lasts more than three hours a day, occurring on more than three days in any week, for three weeks or longer

(Pauli-Pott, Becker, Mertesacker, & Beckmann, 2000). There is some evidence that colic or persistent infant crying can extend even past the first three months (Wolke, Rizzo, & Woods, 2002).

In a study of women from England, New Zealand, and Australia, Kitzinger (1990) gathered a sample of 1,400 women. Out of these, she drew a sample of 100 women whose babies cried the most (more than six hours a day) and 100 women whose babies cried the least (less than two hours a day). Not surprisingly, she found striking differences in the two groups: 80 percent of mothers of babies who cried the most were depressed (compared to 33 percent of mothers whose babies cried the least), 57 percent described a desperate need to escape (compared to 22 percent), 50 percent were "itching" to smack the baby (compared to 20 percent), and 33 percent made negative comments about their partners (compared to 4 percent). Common themes included feeling trapped, that they could not get away, and that they felt guilty, useless, exhausted, inadequate, and bewildered.

Similarly, Pauli-Pott et al. (2000) found that even when babies did not meet Wessel criteria, mothers were significantly more likely to feel angry and nervous and to believe that babies cried because they were dissatisfied with their mothers. Mothers in this study appeared to have great difficulty tolerating their babies' crying and handling their babies. These mothers often felt rejected by their babies, and the mothers reacted with anger and disappointment.

Persistent crying in infancy may also be related to problems later on. In a prospective study of sixty-four infants referred for persistent crying, Wolke et al. (2002) followed up with them at eight to ten years of age and compared them to a matched sample of sixty-four classmates. At follow-up, 19 percent of the children referred for persistent crying had hyperactivity problems, compared with only 2 percent of the control children. Parents, and the children themselves, reported more conduct problems. Parents of the persistent criers rated their children's temperaments as more negative, difficult, and demanding. The academic achievement of persistent criers was significantly lower than that of the control children. This was especially true for those with hyperactivity. There was no difference in current depression for mothers.

Infant Sleep

Temperament has also been shown to influence infant sleep. In a study of forty-one full-term newborns, sleep patterns were recorded for the first two days of life. They were then followed up at eight months, at which time their mothers completed a measure of infant temperament. The infants were grouped into four groups: easy, intermediate, difficult, and most difficult. The sleep measures collected on days 1 and 2 differed significantly between the four groups (Novosad, Freudigman, & Thoman, 1999). Babies rated as difficult had the most disturbed sleep as newborns.

Depression-Related Distortions

An issue that frequently arises in the study of infant temperament is whether the difficulties are real or simply a matter of depressed mothers seeing their children in a more negative light (Najman et al., 2000). Mothers' mental representations of their infants can influence how they interpret their infants' behaviors and, in turn, their response to their infants. This can influence how settled their babies are. A study from Sweden (Canivet et al., 2002) found a subgroup of infants who were genuinely colicky by objective measure. Interestingly, women who indicated, during late pregnancy, that there was a risk of spoiling a baby with too much contact were more likely to have a colicky baby. Infants of these mothers were more distressed, even when given the same amount of physical contact as other babies.

In one study (Rosenblum, McDonough, Muzik, Miller, & Sameroff, 2002), mothers' beliefs about their infants had an impact on infant affect regulation over and above the impact of maternal depression. Rosenblum et al. also found that mothers with distorted representations of their infants were more likely to also report depressive symptoms.

In a study comparing depressed and nondepressed women, the depressed women had more overall negative perceptions of caring for their infants but did not perceive them as temperamentally difficult. Rather, they tended to blame themselves for their infants' behaviors. This was despite the fact that independent raters determined that the infants were in reality more difficult (Whiffen & Gotlib, 1989). The mothers' depression was related to the infants' negative behaviors, which was likely to exacerbate the mothers' negative mood.

In another study, mothers' ratings of infant temperament were related to attachment. Mothers who described their infants as difficult at four months were less likely to have securely attached infants at twelve months. Furthermore, mothers who perceived their infants as difficult tended to have more aversive reactions to an infant's crying (as measured by physiological criteria) and were more likely to use punitive child-rearing techniques (Frodi, Bridges, & Shonk, 1989).

Whiffen (1990) asked mothers to rate their children's temperament two years after participating in a study on postpartum depression. She also assessed the mother's current level of depression. Whiffen found that the correlation between postpartum depression and infant temperament was accounted for by mothers' current level of depression. Agreement of ratings of mothers and fathers were only somewhat consistent, and more disagreement tended to occur when mothers were depressed.

Mothers' Perceptions of Older Children

Depression, and its influence on mothers' perceptions of their children, lasts well past infancy. Maternal depression led to negative biases in reporting children's symptoms of attention-deficit/hyperactivity disorder (ADHD), general behavior problems, and their own negative parenting styles, compared with laboratory assessment, in a sample of ninety-six six- to ten-year-olds (Chi & Hinshaw, 2002).

Mothers who were depressed or anxious were also more likely to report behavior problems in their children at fourteen years of age (Najman et al., 2000). There was a systematic difference in the way mothers reported on the behavior of their children. Since no outside verification of the children's behavior was used in this study (such as teacher or friend report), the authors had no way of knowing whether the children actually did have more behavior problems. The authors suggested that mothers who are depressed may have more difficulties in coping with their children's behaviors and may perceive them as more negative across the board.

In summary, infants with difficult temperaments can have a negative impact on their mothers' emotional state. But a mother's depression can also influence how she sees her child's behavior. An intervention that addresses depression and gives mothers tools to cope with the behavior of their children is likely to be the most effective.

INFANT HEALTH ISSUES

My first child was premature. He was born at thirty-five weeks with severe hyaline membrane disease. . . . He was in the hospital for five months; in the NICU for four months and in intermediate care for one month. . . . The depression started around the time he was three or four weeks old. . . . Up until that time, everything had been so urgent. He had had a couple of arrests. It was overwhelming. Suddenly my son was doing better. Why was I feeling so bad? I had difficulties going to sleep. I was up several times during the night. It was difficult to wake up in the morning. I didn't want to do anything during the day except sleep and call the NICU to check in. I started not to eat well. I felt an impending sense of doom. The depression lasted about a month. . . . About a month after he came home, I felt physically depressed, same as in the initial postpartum period. I brought home a very sick baby. I think it was a delayed reaction, reliving the early part. (Patricia)

Infants with health problems can also influence their mothers' emotional state. Yet postpartum depression is often overlooked in women whose babies are not healthy. It is important that we do not overlook depression because feelings from the postpartum period can have a long-term impact on how a mother copes, how she sees her child, and her level of attachment.

Prematurity

The birth of a premature infant precipitates a psychological crisis. Women who give birth to a premature infant must face the reality of an infant who may be sickly or fragile when they themselves are psychologically and physically depleted. Mothers may experience guilt for an early delivery or anxiety regarding the viability and morbidity of their infants. The babies may also be born following a difficult pregnancy or an emergency delivery. Some of the aspects of medical care of a premature or sick newborn may contribute to the mother's grief and depression. Jan, who had a very difficult pregnancy and delivery, described her feelings after the birth of her daughter. Her daughter was delivered six weeks premature, via emergency cesarean section, after Jan developed eclampsia.

They took her away right after delivery. I never got to hold her, after all that [the difficult pregnancy and delivery]. They brought her back, but my arms were tied to the delivery table. I wish they had released at least one arm. It was really hard.... Leaving the hospital without the baby was really bad. I left early because I didn't want to leave at eleven a.m. with all the other moms and babies.... I shouldn't complain because she only had a few preemie problems. Others in the nursery were so sick. But it was very stressful. It was awful to see them putting the feeding tube down her throat, hearing her gagging and crying. It makes me cry now just to think about it.

Depression can happen at many different times throughout an infant's illness. Mothers may be particularly at risk immediately following delivery, after any medical crisis, when the mother must leave the hospital without the baby, when the baby is about to be discharged, or after the baby is home. A mother's risk of depression is further increased if the baby is transferred to another hospital, particularly if the hospital is in another city. If mothers follow their babies to these other hospitals, they may be cut off from their normal support systems, including their partners.

In some cases, especially with babies who are very sick, mothers may experience anticipatory grieving, and begin to mourn the loss of their infants. In this process, they may distance themselves from their babies in order to prepare themselves for their babies' eventual death. When babies recover, this process of mourning is interrupted, and mothers have to readjust.

Severity of Illness

The severity of illness for premature babies varies widely, ranging from mild to life threatening. Some babies are hospitalized for only a few days, while others may be in intensive care for several weeks or months. Blumberg (1980) examined the direct relationship between neonatal illness and maternal depression. She hypothesized that the greater the degree of neonatal risk, the more depressed the mothers would be. She collected data from 100 postpartum women whose infants had a variety of neonatal conditions. Risk was coded on a five-point scale ("none" to "highest"). Blumberg's results revealed that neonatal risk was significantly correlated with depression: the higher the risk, the greater the depression. Infant risk alone accounted for a significant amount of the variance in depression. Mothers with babies who were most at risk had higher levels of anxiety and more negative perceptions of their newborns than did mothers whose babies were not at risk. This sample was ethnically and demographically diverse, indicating that the effects of neonatal risk were independent of other characteristics within the sample.

Mandated bed rest during pregnancy can also make mothers feel that their babies are at high risk (Maloni, Kane, Suen, & Wang, 2002). In this study, sixty-three women were admitted to hospitals for antepartum bed rest. Dysphoria was related to obstetric risk. Women whose pregnancies had the highest risk scores had the highest levels of dysphoria. Gestational age and health of the baby at birth were significantly correlated with postpartum dysphoria.

In a study of thirty mothers of premature babies, ways of coping, knowledge of infant development, and ways mothers used to gain information were all related to depressive symptoms (Veddovi, Kenny, Gibson, Bowen, & Starte, 2001). Mothers who used informal ways of gaining information about infants (e.g., via other mothers), who used more avoidance coping, and who had less accurate information about infant development were significantly more likely to become depressed. These three variables accounted for 48 percent of the variance in maternal depression.

Mother-Baby Interactions

Premature babies can be very unpredictable in their daily patterns, and this can be taxing for parents (Boukydis, Lester, & Hoffman, 1987). They may also be overly sensitive to stimulation and not as responsive as full-term babies. Because these babies may not be as responsive as normal babies, mothers may overstimulate them, causing the infants to withdraw even further. The mothers may respond to this withdrawal by either increasing the amount of stimulation or withdrawing from the baby, thus creating a vicious cycle (Jarvis, Myers, & Creasey, 1989).

Jarvis et al. (1989) compared three groups of premature infants: those with no medical complications, those who were moderately ill (respiratory distress syndrome), and those who were very ill (bronchopulmonary dysplasia) at four and eight months of age. As predicted, degree of illness did influence the mother-infant interaction at two time points. Mothers of the sickest infants were less sensitive to their infants' cues, did not respond well to their infants' distress, and did not foster social-emotional growth compared with mothers in the other two groups. Moreover, mothers of the sickest infants became less responsive to their infants over time, perhaps reflecting their increasing withdrawal. In contrast, mothers of the moderately ill infants actually became more sensitive in their responses over this same time period.

Long-Term Health Problems

Low birth weight and prematurity can also lead to other problems in children, including ongoing health problems and chronic conditions. In one study, low birth weight was related to the development of ADHD. In this study (Mick, Biederman, Prince, Fischer, & Faraone, 2002), 252 children with ADHD were compared with 231 children without ADHD. The results indicated that children with ADHD were three times more likely to have had low birth weight than the comparison children. These findings held even after controlling for prenatal exposure to alcohol and cigarettes, parental ADHD, social class, and comorbid disruptive behavior of family members. Low birth weight appears to be an independent risk factor for ADHD, but children with low birth weight are a relatively small percentage of children with ADHD.

Kangaroo Care

One technique that can be useful for mothers of premature infants is kangaroo care. The story of kangaroo care is quite amazing. Developed by two neonatologists in Bogotá, Colombia—Drs. Rey and Martinez—it was a solution born of desperation. Before kangaroo care, the mortality rate for premature babies in Colombia was 70 percent. Sanitation in the hospital was often poor. Babies often had to share incubators. Electricity was sporadic or nonexistent. Hospital buildings were rarely heated. Many mothers coped with this situation by abandoning their babies.

Once kangaroo care was implemented, the mortality rate dropped to 30 percent, and the percentage of mothers who abandoned their babies was near zero (Ludington-Hoe, 1993). Kangaroo care has been adopted in many regions of the world, including some hospitals in the United States.

Kangaroo care involves placing the baby, wearing only a diaper, between the mother's breasts or on one breast, under her clothing. The babies are held in a sling or pouch. Fathers can also do kangaroo care. The benefits for babies appear almost immediately. They are calmer. Their body temperature is stable. They cry less, thereby conserving precious calories. The babies do better physically and are discharged from the hospital earlier. Mothers also benefit. They feel more confident in caring for their babies and are more likely to form a secure attachment (Anderson, 1991).

In a case study, Dombrowski, Anderson, Santori, and Burkhammer (2001) found that kangaroo care was helpful for a mother at high risk for depression. She was twenty-two years old, single, and had given up a previous baby for adoption. State agencies removed her and her brother from their home when she was five because of repeated physical and sexual abuse by her father. She and her brother were adopted at age nine after four years in multiple foster homes. She had an active history of substance abuse. Immediately after her baby's premature birth, she was severely depressed. However, within twenty-four hours of starting kangaroo care, she was no longer depressed. She was assessed at six weeks, three months, and seven months, and was neither depressed nor abusing substances at any of these assessments. In describing her experience, she noted the following:

> It was important to both of us for bonding. It made me feel closer than I felt holding her regular, you know, wrapped. It calmed her down a lot more and made her more secure. It made me close to her and I was scared to be a mother but it gave me a sense of peace that I could do it [take care of the baby]. It made me less stressed and able to relax—a "time out" together kind of thing. I was able to forget everything else. It worked well for both of us on stress. I felt like I needed something and being a recovering drug addict I needed this to help. (Dombrowski et al., 2001, p. 215)

A study from Israel showed similar results with a larger sample (Feldman, Eidelman, Sirota, & Weller, 2002). This study randomly assigned preterm infants to either kangaroo care or standard care. The mothers were matched according to infants' birth weight, gestational age, medical problem severity, and demographics. At thirty-seven weeks gestation, mothers in the kangaroo care group had more positive affect, touch, and adaptation to their infants' cues. The infants showed more alertness and less gaze aversion. The mothers were less likely to be depressed and to report that their infants were abnormal. At three months, mothers and fathers were more sensitive and provided a better home environment (based on score on the Home Observation for Measurement of the Environment [HOME] inventory). At six months, the kangaroo care mothers were more sensitive to their babies' cues, and their infants scored significantly higher on the Bayley Mental Developmental Index and the Psychomotor Developmental Index. The authors speculated that kangaroo care influenced infant development directly by having a positive impact on infants' perceptual-cognitive and motor development. It may also have had an indirect impact because kangaroo care improved maternal mood, mothers' perceptions of their infants, and their interactive behavior. In another study, kangaroo care was related to successful lactation in mothers of very low birth weight infants, even after controlling for maternal age, race, marital status, and education beyond high school (Furman, Minich, & Hack, 2002).

Even with nonpremature infants, infant carrying can be a useful strategy. In a sample of low-income mothers of newborns, researchers randomly assigned them to either baby carriers (more contact) or infant seat (less contact) conditions (Anisfeld, Casper, Nozyce, & Cunningham, 1990). At two months, 52 percent of the control infants had a daily period of crying, whereas only 21 percent of the experimental infants did so. At three months, mothers in the baby carrier condition were more contingently responsive to their babies' vocalizations. At thirteen months, mothers in the carrier condition were significantly more likely to be securely attached to their infants. The carrying technique did not have an impact on infant temperament, however. Interestingly, significantly fewer mothers had avoidant babies in the experimental group (13 percent versus 39 percent). Previous studies have found that mothers of avoidant infants often have a physical aversion to contact with their babies. The authors concluded that carrying babies may have helped mothers overcome these feelings, and concluded that using a soft baby carrier makes mothers more responsive to their infants and promotes secure attachment.

Prematurity is only one type of health issue that can influence mothers. Infants' long-term health problems, such as disability and chronic illness, can also affect mothers. Studies of this issue are described in the next section.

Disability or Chronic Illness

Disabilities also vary considerably in their impairment of a child's functioning and how they impact mothers. In a sample from India, infant hospital admission was highly significantly associated with postpartum depression (Patel et al., 2002). Similarly, serious infant health problems were a risk factor for Turkish women at six months postpartum (Danaci et al., 2002). Even relatively minor problems can lead to mothers being separated from their babies and can cause considerable emotional pain.

Long-Term Effects of Infant/Child Illness

Chronic health problems in infants can influence mothers at several levels. They can trigger grief reactions and make mothers vulnerable to depression. Infant illness can also influence the mother-infant interaction. In a study of atopic dermatitis (AD; Pauli-Pott, Darui, & Beckman, 1999), three groups of mothers were compared: those with three- to four-month-olds with AD, those with ten- to twelve-month-olds with AD, and those with healthy infants. Mothers of infants with AD described themselves as more depressed and hopeless. They were more anxious and overprotective. They characterized their infants as less frequently positive and more frequently negative than infants in the control group.

Fischer-Fay, Goldberg, Simmons, and Levison (1988) compared fifteen-month-old infants with cystic fibrosis (CF) to healthy infants of the same age. The results revealed no differences in attachment patterns for infants with CF and healthy infants. However, within the group of CF infants, those with the lowest weights were significantly more likely to have insecure attachments to their mothers. Another study (Williamson, Walters, & Shaffer, 2002) found that a negative model of self and others predicted depression in mothers of children with chronic pain. Maternal depression and child self-reported pain also predicted depression in their children. A mother's avoidance of other people and the situation was a critical factor in how well she coped with her child's illness.

A study of mothers of children with epilepsy also demonstrated the relationship between children's illness and mothers' depression (Mu, Wong, Chang, & Kwan, 2001). The children in this study ranged in age from one to nineteen years. The authors found three factors associated with maternal depression: boundary ambiguity, uncertainty, and mother's age, with younger mothers having more difficulty coping with their children's illness. These three factors accounted for 21 percent of the variance in maternal depression. Uncertainty refers to inadequate ability to structure or categorize an event due to lack of sufficient cues. Epilepsy by nature is difficult to predict. Boundary ambiguity refers to an uncertain role of the child in the family. Because of the illness, parents are unsure what role their children can fulfill. For example, should they be assigned household chores? Caretakers may be either inadequately or excessively involved.

Similarly, mothers' feelings that they could not manage their children's asthma increased the likelihood of hospitalization for asthma (Chen, Bloomberg, Fisher, & Strunk, 2003). In this study, 115 children (ages four to eighteen) were followed for a year. All the children had at least one hospitalization during the study period. If parents thought they could do nothing to manage their children's asthma, or if they felt overwhelmed by caring for their children, their children were more likely to be hospitalized for acute attacks. This effect was found even after controlling for baseline severity of asthma, medications, and child age. Some other characteristics related to increased hospitalization included greater levels of family strain and conflict and greater financial strain.

The total amount of stress a woman faces can also influence her attentiveness. Birth order interacted with degree of prematurity and illness in one study (Bendersky & Lewis, 1986). As predicted, primiparous women were more attentive to the needs of their high-risk infants than mothers whose high-risk infants were later born. The results of this study most likely reflect the increased burdens of having to care both for an older healthy child (or children) and a later-born high-risk infant.

The results of these studies, and the comments of the mothers I have spoken with, indicate that infants with health problems can be taxing for parents and can also be related to maternal depression. In some cases, women may resent the extra burdens their infants place on the family. They may also feel guilty for these feelings and withdraw from others. It is during this phase that social support for mothers is crucial. In the next section, I review research that has specifically addressed the issue of social support for mothers of infants with health issues.

Social Support for Mothers of Infants with Health Issues

I found it difficult to speak with my husband and family about being depressed, and about my constant concern and worry. They kept trying to be positive, saying what they would do with him when he got well. I don't know if my medical knowledge made it worse. I knew how serious it was. It made me more depressed when my family was upbeat and tried to deny how serious it was. I had to deal with their denial and I felt they were heaping expectations on me. . . . I got lots of support from a couple we're friends with. She's an NICU nurse. They would offer to sit at the hospital for us so we could go out. They also made meals for us. They were people who understood the medical issues. They didn't say everything would be okay. They realized it could be fatal. (Patricia)

Social support can mediate many of the negative effects of having a baby with a health problem. It can take many forms, including information, practical assistance, and emotional support. The results of two studies indicated that social support can positively affect attachment between mothers and at-risk infants. In the first study, mothers of infants with disabilities initially showed fewer attachment behaviors at one month postpartum than did the comparison group of mothers of nondisabled babies, regardless of the length of hospital stay (Capuzzi, 1989). By six and twelve months, however, these differences had disappeared. Social support for the mother reduced the stress of having a child with a disability and facilitated attachment. The author suggested that attachment is a dynamic process that develops over time. Although mothers of infants with disabilities may have a more difficult time developing this attachment, they can adapt and develop it. Similar results were found in a study of fifty-two high-risk premature infants (Crnic, Greenberg, & Slough, 1986).

Social support has also been helpful in facilitating attachment and infant development in babies identified as being at-risk because of maternal depression and poverty (Lyons-Ruth, Connell, Grunebaum, & Botein, 1990). In this study, thirty depressed mothers were given weekly home visiting services. They were compared with depressed mothers of similar low socioeconomic status at eighteen months. The home-visiting services provided information and emotional support and overcame the effects of maternal depression for the infants. Those who received these services had infants with scores an average of ten points higher on the Bayley Scales, and were twice as likely to be classified as securely attached. The authors did not report whether the mothers who received services were less depressed, however.

Another study (Affleck, Tennen, Rowe, Roscher, & Walker, 1989) indicated that formal social support for mothers of high-risk babies is only effective if the mothers perceive a need for support. When the mothers needed support, the program (consisting of support and information from in-home nurse consultants) improved mothers' sense of perceived control, competence, and responsiveness. The program had a negative effect on mothers who had a low perceived need for support, by actually making them feel less competent and more anxious. This was a surprising finding. To explain it, the authors took a closer look at the interaction between the home visitors and mothers in this group. They found that since these mothers did not feel they needed services, the home visitors were trying to convince them that they did. Not surprisingly, the mothers felt more anxious after receiving this type of "support."

CONCLUSION

Both mothers and at-risk babies bring special challenges to the mother-infant relationship. Mothers may be in the process of grieving when they are forced to deal with babies who are different from what they expected and who may be difficult to handle. In spite of these difficulties, attachment can develop between mother and baby, especially if the mother is given adequate support (and she perceives it as support). You can do much to facilitate these types of positive reactions. Helping mothers feel competent in caring for their at-risk babies is vital for reducing risk for postpartum depression and helping mothers to become attached to their babies.

In the next chapter, I describe psychological risk factors for postpartum depression.

Chapter 6

Psychological Risk Factors

Psychosocial influences are a common explanation for postpartum depression. Professionals who do not attribute postpartum depression to biological factors are likely to attribute it to unrealistic expectations or lack of support. Because this is such a large category, I have divided it into psychological and social risk factors. In this chapter, I describe the psychological factors. Social factors are described in Chapter 7.

The psychological factors include a woman's attributional style; her expectations about what it will be like to be a mother; her self-esteem; how competent she feels as a parent; and prior vulnerability factors such as loss, previous psychiatric illness, and a dysfunctional or abusive family history.

ATTRIBUTIONAL STYLE

I hadn't handled a lot of babies. The nurse was yelling at me, saying, "What's the matter, haven't you handled a baby before?" I was offended and hurt. All I could think of was, "I'm a bad mother." . . . When [the depression] was really bad, I thought, "I'm a bad person. I should have never had a baby, never gotten married. I'm a bad mother. I'm crap." I talked about it all the time until others were sick of hearing about it. . . . At one point, my mom said to me, "I don't know what you are worried about. One baby is no work." All I could think was, "I'm a failure." (Barbara)

In describing how people see the world, we might refer to them as optimists or pessimists. Researchers use the term *attributional style* to encompass both. A pessimistic attributional style predicts vulnerability to depression following stress because people who have this style have learned to interpret events in a way that makes them more stressful and negative. People with a pessimistic style see events as outside of their control and believe that they cannot change negative aspects of their lives.

In a reformulation of the learned-helplessness model, Abramson, Seligman, and Teasdale's (1978) classic paper identified three components of the depression-prone (pessimistic) attributional style. Specifically, pessimists are more likely to become depressed after a negative event because they maintain internal, global, and stable attributions about why negative events occurred. Internal attributions mean that the cause of the negative event is within the person's control. Negative events can also be attributed to stable ("I am stupid") or unstable ("I was tired") characteristics. Global attributions mean that people feel that negative events affect many areas of their lives, while persons who make specific attributions realize that negative events only affect one or two areas.

Although this research refers to depression in general, attributional style has also been studied in relation to depression in new mothers. An Australian study of sixty-five primiparous women found that dysfunctional attitudes were related to depression at six weeks postpartum. This was especially true for women with high amounts of postpartum stress and for women whose babies had difficult temperaments (Grazioli & Terry, 2000). Negative thinking and thoughts of death and dying at one month postpartum predicted depression at four months in a study of 465 postpartum women (Chaudron et al., 2001). The authors considered thoughts of dying as a prodrome of later depression. Interestingly, although women who breastfed their infants did not differ from women who bottle-fed in the development of depression, women who worried about breastfeeding were significantly more likely to become depressed than those who did not worry.

Optimism was found to influence birth outcomes in a medically high-risk sample of 129 women (Lobel, DeVincent, Kaminer, & Meyer, 2000). In this study, prenatal stress and optimism were examined in relation to birth outcomes (birth weight and gestational age), controlling for risk and ethnicity. Using structural equation modeling, the authors found that women who were less optimistic had babies who weighed significantly less even when controlling for gestational age. Prenatal stress did not have an effect once optimism was added to the model. Some of this difference may have been behavioral. Optimists were more likely to exercise, and exercise lowered the risk of preterm birth.

Donovan and colleagues (Donovan & Leavitt, 1989; Donovan, Leavitt, & Walsh, 1990) examined attributional style through the construct "illusory control." Subjects who had high illusory control were those who reported that they had control over events that were, in reality, beyond their control. In a study of sixty-six mothers of five-month-olds (Donovan et al., 1990), women with high illusory control felt incompetent as parents and were more likely to withdraw from parenting situations. Many of these women experienced guilt when they could not be "perfect mothers." The authors speculated that this attributional style might lead to the overcontrolling and interfering behaviors that appear among depressed mothers of toddlers. In another study of forty-eight mothers of five-month-olds (Donovan & Leavitt, 1989), women with high illusory control were the most depressed and reported the father as participating the least in child care activities. To summarize, women with the high illusory control attributional style were most susceptible to learned helplessness and subsequent depression. When the women found they could not control the events they thought they could, they tended to give up and withdraw from the task.

Control appears to be a factor in both positive and negative attributional styles. When people think they can control events that are indeed controllable, they are optimists. When people think they have no control over events that they can control (learned helplessness) or that they have control over events that they cannot possibly control (high illusory control), they are likely to become depressed. The key appears to be learning to make realistic assessments about which events are controllable and which are not.

SELF-EFFICACY, SELF-ESTEEM, AND EXPECTATIONS

The truth of the matter is that I'm ashamed. Why is it so hard for me and looks so easy for other mothers? I saw other full-time mothers always doing things better. I felt I couldn't keep up. I used to be able to "run with the guys." . . . Now, I'm in a traditional mommy role, but I'm not relating to this role. So where does this leave me? Not fitting into either role. . . . I'm used to being the best at what I do. But I felt I couldn't [function as a mother]. Especially when I look at other moms. I can't seem to understand why I can't do this. . . . I was depending on other people's expectations. Maybe even my own expectations were too high. This led to feeling down, out of control. That's when the depression really started. Doubting I could do it. It got to where I was scared to death, nervous, chest tightness, crying, not wanting to eat.

Self-esteem, self-efficacy, and expectations are three concepts that refer to a woman's adjustment to her role as a mother, what she expects of herself, and how competent she feels. These concepts are closely related and tend to interact. According to Cutrona and Troutman (1986), mothers who have high self-esteem and a high perception of their own self-efficacy tend to be persistent, to avoid making internal attributions for their failures, and to experience less anxiety and depression. On the other hand, those with low self-esteem and a low sense of self-efficacy tend to give up in the face of difficulties, make internal attributions for their failures, and experience high levels of both anxiety and depression. Expectations about what mothers are "supposed" to do influence how a woman evaluates the job she is doing and whether she will feel good about herself in her new role.

Self-Efficacy

Self-efficacy refers to how competent a mother feels in her role and can also influence whether she becomes depressed. In one study, low self-efficacy, as reflected in reports of feeling overwhelmed by child care, was associated with depression severity at two months postpartum (Campbell et al., 1992).

In another study, maternal self-efficacy acted as a mediator between infant temperament and postpartum depression in a study of fifty-five married women. Women who had infants with difficult temperaments felt less competent as mothers and had higher levels of postpartum depression. Social support buffered this effect by increasing self-efficacy and helping the women feel more competent (Cutrona & Troutman, 1986).

Self-Esteem

Self-esteem has also been directly linked to postpartum depression. In a study of eighty postpartum women (Affonso & Arizmendi, 1986), a woman's view of herself and her future was significantly related to whether she was likely to be depressed. The key elements were "not feeling good about myself," "not managing roles well," "future does not look promising," "feel unattractive," and "predominant mood not positive." These items were all significantly and positively correlated with depression.

In a meta-analysis of eighty-four studies, Beck (2001) found that self-esteem had a moderate effect on postpartum depression. Low self-esteem at one month postpartum predicted depression at four months in another study of 465 women (Chaudron et al., 2001). A prospective study of 191 low-income, inner-city women found that self-esteem was related to lower levels of depression in both the prenatal and postpartum periods (Ritter, Hobfoll, Lavin, Cameron, & Hulsizer, 2000).

Expectations

In a metasynthesis of eighteen qualitative studies, Beck (2002) found that expectations played a large role in postpartum depression at several different levels. Beck described how both mothers and professionals who care for them still harbor the belief that motherhood brings total fulfillment to women. Motherhood certainly can be a wonderful experience. But the expectation of total fulfillment from this role, without acknowledging the difficulties, sets standards that are impossible to meet. Women often try to be perfect mothers, and when motherhood turns out to be different than they expected, they feel that they have failed. Women in these studies often did not confide in others because they believed that no one else ever felt that way; they believed they were abnormal mothers. Beck noted that first-time mothers were more prone to the myth of the perfect mother, whereas multiparous women's expectations focused on trying to cope with the new addition to their families.

Expectations of self can also be related to the expression of goals. In a Finnish study (Salmela-Aro, Nurmi, Saisto, & Halmesmaki, 2001), an increase in goals for self ("to grow as a person," "develop myself," or "promote my mental growth") led to an increase in depressive symptoms for women making the transition to motherhood. Conversely, an increase in family-related goals predicted a decrease in depression. Family-related goals included "take good care of my children" or "take good care of my family." When mothers adjusted their personal goals to the demands of the transition to motherhood, their depression declined. The ability to adapt goals to fit within current constraints and resources is an important component of mental health. The authors noted that when people cannot adapt their goals, depression is the likely consequence. Women in this study were assessed during early pregnancy, at eight months gestation, and at three months and two years postpartum.

Women's expectations about their babies can also lead to depression. In a sample of sixty-eight at-risk African-American women, those who worried about spoiling their babies reported more depression and had more inappropriate developmental expectations of their babies than mothers who were less worried about spoiling. These findings suggested that fear of spoiling may influence maternal responsiveness in mothers who are at risk and may lead to potentially disturbed mother-infant relationships (Smyke, Boris, & Alexander, 2002).

In summary, women are more likely to experience postpartum depression if they have unrealistic expectations of themselves as mothers and of their babies. If they have low self-esteem and feel incompetent as mothers, they are also more likely to be depressed.

PREVIOUS PSYCHIATRIC HISTORY

Previous psychiatric history also increases the risk of postpartum depression. Psychiatric history of women or their first-degree relatives was significantly related to whether they would become depressed postpartum in three studies (Campbell et al., 1992; O'Hara, Neunaber, & Zekoski, 1984; Watson, Elliot, Rugg, & Brough, 1984). O'Hara et al. (1984) also found that number of previous episodes of depression increased the risk for postpartum depression.

More recently, Webster, Linnane, Dibley, and Pritchard (2000) compared 600 women with prenatal risk factors for postpartum depression and 301 women without risk factors in their development of depression sixteen weeks after birth. Some 26 percent of the women with risk factors became depressed compared to 11 percent of the control group—2.5 times more. Among the risk factors, a woman's history of psychiatric disorders and a history of postpartum depression were both significantly related to depression. In contrast to previous studies, a family history of mood disorder and a woman's own mother having postpartum depression were not related to the development of depression. Another study found that for women who had an episode of depression at any other point in their lives, their risk of postpartum depression rose to 25 percent (Moline, Kahn, Ross, Altshuler, & Cohen, 2001). In an Irish sample, 29 percent of mothers in a disadvantaged Dublin neighborhood were depressed. Previous treatment for depression was one of four risk factors that strongly predicted depression in this population (Cryan et al., 2001). Previous psychiatric history of the mother or her spouse also predicted the development of postpartum depression in a sample of 257 women from Turkey at six months postpartum (Danaci et al., 2002).

Depression During Pregnancy

Researchers have also found that depression in pregnancy is a risk factor for postpartum depression. Spinelli (1998) describes how antepartum depression is frequently underdiagnosed, even though approximately 10 percent of pregnant women meet criteria for major or minor depression. The risk factors for depression during pregnancy include a personal or family history of depression, previous or current abuse, marital dysfunction, young age, and an increased number of children.

In a large study ($N = 9,028$), depression was measured at eighteen and thirty-two weeks gestation, and at eight weeks and eight months postpartum (Evans, Heron, Francomb, Oke, & Golding, 2001). The authors found that depression rates were highest at thirty-two weeks gestation and lowest at eight months postpartum. They suggested that depression is more likely during pregnancy than it is postpartum. Similarly, Hobfoll, Ritter, Lavin, Hulsizer, and Cameron (1995; Ritter et al., 2000) found the highest percentage of women were depressed during pregnancy. The rates were 28 percent (Time 1) and 25 percent (Time 2) antepartum, and 23 percent postpartum in a sample of 192 low-income women from the inner city. Depression during pregnancy was a weak but significant risk factor for depression postpartum. Only 47 percent of the women with postpartum depression did not have prepartum depression.

In a sample of 252 mothers from India, 23 percent had postpartum depression. But 78 percent of these women were also depressed during pregnancy. Only 21 percent developed depression for the first time during the postpartum period, when they were assessed at six weeks postpartum. Also, 59 percent of women depressed at six weeks were still depressed at six months postpartum (Patel et al., 2002). A study of 465 women found that depression during pregnancy was one of four predictors of depression at four months postpartum (Chaudron et al., 2001).

In a sample of eighty women, 25 percent experienced depression during pregnancy, and 16 percent experienced depression at four to five weeks postpartum (Da Costa, Larouche, Dritsa, & Brender, 2000). Women who were depressed postpartum reported more emotional coping and higher state and trait anxiety during pregnancy. The best predictor of postpartum depressed mood was depressed mood during pregnancy. In a low-income minority sample ($N = 802$), 37 percent of the women had depressive symptoms and 6.5 to 8.5 percent had major depression at three to five weeks postpartum. In this sample, 50 percent were also depressed during pregnancy (Yonkers et al., 2001).

In a meta-analysis of eighty-four studies, Beck (2001) found that prenatal depression, prenatal anxiety, and a history of previous depression were all risk factors for postpartum depression with moderate effect sizes ranging from .38 to .46. Similarly, a meta-analysis by O'Hara and Swain (1996) found that depression and anxiety during pregnancy and a mother's history of psychopathology were moderate to strong predictors of postpartum depression.

Previous episodes of depression increase the risk for depression postpartum. The findings are more mixed when describing depression in first-degree relatives. I frequently speak with mothers who are concerned about having a repeat occurrence. We should recognize that an earlier episode or an episode in a family member are risk factors, but do not make depression inevitable. Mothers in this situation should alert their caregivers during pregnancy, arrange for follow-up postpartum, and get extra help and support so they do not exhaust themselves after their babies are born. Recognizing risk and taking steps to counter it can often prevent a recurrence.

VIOLENCE AGAINST WOMEN

Violence against women is a potent pathogen for women's physical and mental health. It includes childhood physical and sexual abuse, rape and sexual assault, and domestic violence, and is related to depression in women. Of all types of violence against women, child sexual abuse has been studied most frequently. Briere and Elliot

(1994) estimated that sexual abuse survivors have a four-time greater lifetime risk for major depression compared with adults who have not been sexually abused. Depression is also common among those who have experienced other types of maltreatment as well.

Depression in Abuse Survivors

In a large representative sample (Nelson et al., 2002), a history of child sexual abuse was related to several serious sequelae including major depression, suicide attempt, alcohol and nicotine dependence, and rape after the age of eighteen. These relationships appeared even after controlling for family background and other risk factors.

Felitti (1991) found that 83 percent of sexually abused patients in a primary care sample were depressed compared with 32 percent of the comparison group. The women's symptoms included sleep disturbances, chronic fatigue, despondency, and frequent crying spells. The majority of the depressed patients had never been treated. In another primary-care sample, women who had been sexually abused were significantly more likely to report feeling blue or depressed. Indeed, 65 percent were depressed, compared with 35 percent of the non-abused group. An even higher percentage (68 percent) reported mood swings, compared with 29 percent of nonabused women. These same women were also more likely to report extreme anger and rage, fear of being alone, and spells of panic or terror (Hulme, 2000).

In a community sample of women, 100 percent of women whose sexual abuse involved penetration were depressed (Cheasty, Clare, & Collins, 1998). The lifetime prevalence of major depression was 86 percent in sexual abuse survivors with PTSD, and 29 percent of these women were currently depressed (Bremner et al., 1997). An additive effect of physical and sexual abuse also appears to occur in depression. According to the results of the Commonwealth Fund Adolescent Health Survey, girls in grades five through twelve who had been both physically and sexually abused were five times more likely to report depressive symptoms and three times more likely to report moderate to high stress than nonabused girls (Diaz, Simatov, & Rickert, 2000).

Exposure to parental violence has also been linked to major depression in a birth cohort sample of eighteen-year-olds from New Zealand: the higher the rate of parental violence, the higher the rate of major depression. The teens in this sample also had a high exposure to both sexual abuse and regular use of physical punishment (Fergusson & Horwood, 1998).

Postpartum Depression in Abuse Survivors

Abuse survivors are also more prone to postpartum depression. Buist and Janson (2001) conducted a three-year follow-up study of mothers who were hospitalized for major depressive disorder during the postpartum period. They discovered that half of these depressed women were sexual abuse survivors. When compared with other depressed women, those who had been abused had higher scores on depression and anxiety measures, and their symptoms showed less improvement over time. The women's partners were also more likely to describe their children as "disturbed." In addition, sexually abused women reported more life stress and had significantly higher scores on the Parenting Stress Index. Val describes how her past history of sexual abuse related to her postpartum depression and how it manifested in obsessional thoughts of harming her twin babies:

My depression started three days after birth. It came on very suddenly. My husband was coming to the hospital. We were going to give the babies a bath. As we were giving [my daughter] a bath, I was suddenly afraid that I might abuse her. I had been sexually abused as a child. I didn't tell anyone until the next day. . . . It started with, "Oh my God. I was abused. I could abuse them." Then it was more general. Everything was a danger. Everything could hurt the kids. . . . I can't tell you how surprised I was. I haven't done anything to hurt the kids. I first visualized my son being thrown into the fire. Then it was me throwing him in. I worried about plastic. I'd have thoughts of smothering the kids with pillows. There were certain rooms in the house I couldn't even go in. I couldn't drink coffee. I'd have thoughts of pouring it on the kids. Through all of this I never neglected my children's needs, no matter how difficult. . . . No one ever questioned that I would hurt the kids. I'm the only one. I feel it could be from the sexual abuse. I obsess and worry about things. I've had times and traumatic events that I've worried about before, but it's always been just me.

The Connection Between Childhood and Domestic Abuse

In her review of the literature, Buist (1998) points out that past abuse appears to make women more vulnerable to current domestic violence, marital strife, divorce, and general mistrust for other people. Each of these can also increase the risk of postpartum depression. In a study of 357 primiparous women, those who had been sexually abused as children were significantly more likely to be depressed during their pregnancies and to have been both physically and verbally abused before and during pregnancy (Benedict, Paine, Paine, Brandt, & Stallings, 1999).

Unfortunately, the combination of past and current abuse can have a devastating impact on women's mental health. Dubowitz et al. (2001) found that when women experienced multiple types of abuse, they were more likely to be depressed, used harsher discipline and parenting, and, not surprisingly, had more problems with their children ($N = 419$). Mothers abused as children and as adults, or who were both physically and sexually abused, had worse outcomes than those who suffered only one type of abuse. Mothers' depression and harsh parenting were directly associated with internalizing and externalizing behavior problems in their children. The authors speculated that mothers who have been victimized might be less attentive to their children and less emotionally available. Moreover, these mothers may have less tolerance for the day-to-day stresses of parenting and may be more inclined to view their children's behaviors as problematic. The authors concluded that a mother's history of victimization appears to be highly prevalent in high-risk samples. More than half of the mothers in their sample had been physically or sexually victimized at some time, and half of the mothers victimized during childhood or adolescence were revictimized as adults.

Parenting Difficulties

As the Dubowitz et al. (2001) study indicates, abuse survivors often have mothering difficulties (Buist, 1998). Some of these difficulties include marital disharmony, lack of parenting consensus, a chaotic family life, low self-confidence, and an insensitivity to their babies' cues. These factors may continue a cycle in which mothers feel inadequate in their new role. They then become angry, frustrated, and depressed in response. Some mothers will respond to these frustrations by becoming abusive or continuing in an abusive relationship that exposes their children to violence. Other mothers will struggle, and while they do not become abusive, their parenting is less than adequate. In a sample of low-income single mothers, childhood abuse and low self-esteem predicted more depressive symptoms (Luten-bacher, 2002). Depression was related to anger. Everyday stressors, when combined with depression, predicted higher levels of anger. But current partner abuse was the best predictor of overall abusive parenting attitudes and parent-child role reversal.

Friedrich and Sims (2003) assessed 391 mothers of children and adolescents who were inpatients at a psychiatric facility. They found that mothers' victimization history was related to lower quality of parenting, reduced satisfaction with social support, greater depression, and more negative attributions about their children. Victimization history included sexual, physical, and emotional abuse. Mothers' victimization history also increased their children's risk of being sexually abused. Not surprisingly, children of these mothers also had high levels of behavior problems, and mothers who experienced multiple types of victimization had children with the most behavioral problems.

Abuse and Breastfeeding

Breastfeeding is also an issue for many abuse survivors. So far, there is little empirical information on how past or current abuse influences a woman's desire and ability to breastfeed. Although not specifically related to depression, this issue can become of central concern for women. Surprisingly, abuse survivors are more likely to want to breastfeed than their nonabused counterparts.

Benedict, Paine, and Paine (1994) studied 360 primiparous women in the Baltimore area. The sample was predominantly African American and low income. Of these women, 12 percent were sexual abuse survivors. A higher percentage of sexual abuse survivors (54 percent) indicated an intention to breastfeed than their nonabused counterparts (41 percent). There were no significant differences between the abuse survivors and nonabused women on rates of cesarean sections, induction or augmentation of labor, anesthesia during labor or birth, or failure to progress.

Prentice, Lu, Lange, and Halfon (2002) had similar findings with a different population of mothers. This study included a national sample of 1,220 mothers with children younger than age three. Of these women, 7 percent indicated that they were survivors of sexual abuse. As with the previous study, women who had been sexually abused were twice as likely to initiate breastfeeding (odds ratio [OR] = 2.58).

In a sample of 212 women recruited from a population of individuals enrolled in the Woman, Infants and Children (WIC) supplemental nutrition program, Bullock, Libbus, and Sable (2001) examined the question of whether women with abuse histories, or those currently being abused, would be less likely to breastfeed their infants. The authors found no relationship between past or current abuse and feeding choice for their infants. The women who suffered from past or current abuse breastfed their infants in the same proportion as those who were not currently being abused.

Some women who are abuse survivors may ask you, even before they become pregnant, whether they will be able to breastfeed. In my experience, the answer is a resounding "it depends." We should not discourage mothers from trying it. But we should also be realistic about some of the difficulties they might encounter (see Kendall-Tackett, 2001, for more specific suggestions on how to avoid some of the difficulties survivors face while breastfeeding). In the following account, abuse survivor Beth Dubois (2003) describes how she was nervous about giving birth and breastfeeding her son. The theme of low self-efficacy is evident. But she also describes how breastfeeding was healing and empowering for her.

> As the time of my son's birth approached, my worries about breastfeeding came into sharp focus. . . . I now see that not only has breastfeeding been possible for me, a survivor of childhood sexual abuse, it has been immensely healing. My desire to have a fulfilling breastfeeding relationship forced me to face emotional territory I would probably have otherwise avoided. One wound left by the abuse is an underlying sense of "I can't do it. It's not even worth trying." Birthing and breastfeeding Theodore has helped to replace this with a very real sense of capability and confidence. (pp. 50-51)

Abuse survivors have a higher lifetime risk for depression than the general population. We should, therefore, not be surprised when they are at increased risk during the postpartum period. As I described for previous psychiatric illness, past abuse is a risk factor for depression. But depression is not inevitable. It can be helpful for mothers to check in with their care providers periodically, as well as any mental health providers that they have seen in the past. You might also want to have a list of referral sources ready for mothers who are dealing with past abuse for the first time in the postpartum period.

LOSS

The final psychological factor I describe is loss. Loss can also predict depression and can take many forms. Loss of a parent during childhood can create a lifetime risk for depression (Watson et al., 1984). Childhood illness and abuse can also represent loss of a "normal" childhood (Gotlib, Whiffen, Wallace, & Mount, 1991). As I described in Chapter 4, childbearing loss can also increase the probability of depression during subsequent pregnancies and after a new baby is born (Hughes et al., 1999). Recent loss of a partner through death or divorce or loss of a parent can also predispose a mother to postpartum depression (see Kendall-Tackett, 2001).

One study examined the long-term effects of parental divorce, later depression, and the subjects' subsequent divorce (O'Connor, Thorpe, Dunn, & Golding, 1999). It found a long-term correlation between parental divorce in childhood and depression in adulthood. This association was partly mediated by the quality of the parent-child relationship, teenage pregnancy, leaving home before age eighteen, and the subject's level of educational attainment.

Loss was also a theme in Beck's (2002) metasynthesis of eighteen qualitative studies. She noted, "loss permeated deep into the crevices of depressed mothers' lives. It insidiously seeped into the very fiber of their beings" (p. 466). Women in these studies described several types of loss. The first was the loss of self. This consisted of two components: loss of current self and loss of a former self. Women did not know who they were after they had their babies and described how they had lost their sexuality, power in the family, personal space, intellectual ability and memory, and occupation. Related to this is loss of identity. This was especially an issue for women who had worked outside the home before they had their babies.

Beck (2002) also described loss of relationships. Women agonized over lost relationships with their infants or other children, partners, friends, and family. They felt depression had robbed them of the positive feelings they should have for their babies. Sometimes women described how they resented and became angry with their babies. Loss of relationships also occurred with women's older children. They suddenly became resentful of their older children's needs and felt that their older children were "suffocating" them. Women's relationships with their partners became strained. Women admitted resenting their partners and wishing that their partners would take the initiative to help them. On the other hand, many were ashamed that they were struggling, because it meant they were inadequate or failures as mothers. These feelings of inadequacy kept them isolated from other mothers, whom they assumed were doing a much better job than they were.

The final loss described by Beck (2002) was loss of voice. Mothers suffering from depression made a conscious effort to silence their own voices. They feared the reaction of others if they admitted how they had been struggling. They did not want to burden friends or family and feared being rejected or misunderstood. One mother described her experience as "imprisoned in my own prison" (p. 468). When they did find their voices, partners or others often did silence or reject them, contributing further to their loss of voice.

CONCLUSION

The studies cited in this chapter demonstrate that how a woman feels about herself, her general outlook on life, and her family history can either protect her or make her vulnerable to depression in the puerperium and beyond. Psychological factors such as prior trauma and loss, a negative attributional style, and unrealistic expectations can all contribute to a mother's risk of depression.

Depression in pregnancy also raises some issues about how we conceptualize postpartum depression. It appears, from this research, that depression during pregnancy is at least as likely as postpartum depression. If that is the case, then it is inaccurate to consider the postpartum period a time of unique vulnerability. On the other hand, it might be useful for us to conceptualize postpartum depression in life-span perspective—to see vulnerability to depression as occurring over the life of a woman, and that both pregnancy and postpartum are vulnerable times.

On a more hopeful note, even with significant risk factors, depression is not inevitable. All of these psychological risk factors can be addressed in therapy. Cognitive therapy, in particular, has been shown to be efficacious in addressing thoughts and beliefs that increase the likelihood of depression (see Chapter 10).

Chapter 7

Social Risk Factors

Women do not become mothers in a vacuum. They live in families, extended families, cultures, and societies. At each of these levels of social connection, mothers can be protected from, or made more vulnerable to, depression. The social factors related to depression include the amount of help a mother has with her baby and other children, the amount of emotional support she receives from her partner and others around her, her socioeconomic status, and her exposure to stressful life events. Each of these is described in this chapter.

STRESSFUL LIFE EVENTS

Life does not stop when a woman becomes pregnant. It goes on. If women experience significant life stresses during pregnancy or the postpartum period, they are more vulnerable to depression. In one study, Chinese women who developed postpartum depression experienced significantly more stressful life events than their nondepressed counterparts (Xu & Lu, 2001). In her meta-analysis, Beck (2001) found that two types of stress (child care and life stress) had a moderate effect on postpartum depression.

Ritter et al. (2000) found that stressful life events were positively correlated with postpartum depression in a sample of 191 low-income women. The stressful life events fell into eight categories: death of a loved one, problems with spouse or partner, economic hardships, problems with friends or family, discrimination, stressful life events related to pregnancy, general life difficulties, and events that caused depression in the past (e.g., death of a parent).

Stressful life events can also take place in the broader community. Dawn describes how the events of September 11, 2001, influenced her and made her vulnerable to depression.

We had a joint baby shower on September 8. September 11 was three days later. My sister was injured, and we couldn't find her for several hours. I was getting bits and pieces of information. I think my depression started then. I didn't get really bad until after delivery. . . . I've been seeing a psychologist, sometimes twice a week. We're dealing with the disappointment with my difficult pregnancy, my birth, the guilt about not being the perfect mother, September 11.

In contrast, O'Hara et al. (1984) found no relation between depression and life events but found significant relationships between other measures of life stress and depression, such as obstetric risk factors and child care stress. They concluded that it is not the gradual accumulation of stressors that causes depression. Rather, it is a series of stressors that occur over a fairly short time. Along these same lines, Cowan and Cowan (1987) observed that it is not the sheer amount of life stress that causes depression but the balance of life stress and available support. When support is inadequate, stressful events have negative effects on young families.

In summary, life events can act as stressors. They are particularly likely to cause postpartum depression when a mother is already vulnerable. Some things that make her vulnerable include a negative attributional style, low self-esteem and self-efficacy, lack of social support, or a combination of these factors.

MATERNAL AGE

Research on the relationship between postpartum depression and maternal age has yielded inconsistent results. But it appears that mothers on the high and low ends of the age spectrum have the highest risk for depression. One recent prospective study of 901 women found that women under the age of twenty were at high risk for postpartum depression (Webster, Linnane, Dibley, & Pritchard, 2000). The high-risk mothers were also significantly more likely to be unmarried and primiparous. Another study of 465 women found that women ages twenty to twenty-four, or thirty and older, were significantly more likely to be depressed at four months postpartum

(Chaudron et al., 2001). At nine months postpartum, mothers over age thirty-four were at increased risk for depression (Astbury et al., 1994). Adolescent mothers reported significantly lower self-esteem, more parenting stress, more child abuse potential, and a poorer quality of home environment than mothers who were not adolescents in another study. Although this study did not address depression, it does demonstrate that the younger mothers are more prone to risk factors for depression (Andreozzi, Flanagan, Seifer, Brunner, & Lester, 2002).

In a large study of U.S. adults ($N = 2,592$), Mirowsky and Ross (2002) compared three groups of young adults: nonparents, those who became parents before age twenty-three, and those who became parents after age twenty-three. They found that respondents who were younger than twenty-three at first birth reported more depression than nonparents. Nonparents were more depressed than respondents whose first birth was after age twenty-three. Women who had their babies at age thirty had the lowest levels of depression.

In summary, mothers at either end of the age spectrum are vulnerable to depression. Young mothers may be more at risk for depression because they have a higher likelihood of single marital status, low socioeconomic status, and possible past abuse (reflected in teen mother status, and/or earlier age of consensual sexual activity). Older mothers may have been through infertility assessments, high-risk pregnancies, and possible pregnancy loss. They may have had multiple babies as a result of fertility treatments. In addition, older mothers have often attained a higher education level and react with shock when mothering is difficult and overwhelming. These mothers often feel that they cannot complain since they went to such great lengths to become pregnant.

SOCIOECONOMIC STATUS

Poverty also increases the likelihood of depression. The American Psychological Association, in its report on women and depression, noted that poverty was an independent risk factor for depression in women (McGrath, Keita, Strickland, & Russo, 1990). Unfortunately, poverty is very much a mothers' issue. According to the U.S. Census Bureau (1998), mothers in female-headed households had the highest rates of poverty of any demographic group and also comprised the majority of poor families. This was not true for households headed by single fathers.

Poverty makes things difficult for new mothers because it limits support, access to medical care, and access to community resources. Poor mothers often face additional stresses as they deal with uncertain income, dangerous housing or neighborhoods, and the negative effects of being at the bottom of the social strata. The connection between poverty and depression has been found in both American and international samples.

American Samples

In a low-income inner-city sample, Hobfoll et al. (1995) found rates of depression (ranging from 23 to 28 percent) that were nearly twice those of middle-class samples during pregnancy and the post-partum period. They considered poverty a significant risk factor for pre- and postpartum depression.

In a study of 114 Hispanic and African-American women with low-risk pregnancies, 51 percent were depressed. The women's depression scores correlated to other health-related variables including bodily pain, general health, and emotional and physical functioning. Interestingly, there was no difference in social support between the depressed and nondepressed women (McKee et al., 2001).

In the National Maternal Health Survey ($N = 7,537$), a stratified nationally representative sample of births in 1988, 23.8 percent were depressed when their babies were approximately seventeen months old. This study sampled from forty-eight states, the District of Columbia, and New York City. Black mothers, low-income mothers, and mothers of low birthweight babies were oversampled (McLennan & Kotelchuck, 2000; McLennan, Kotelchuck, & Cho, 2001). Three years later, 16.6 percent were depressed, and 36 percent of those with elevated depression scores at first survey had elevated depression scores at second survey (McLennan et al., 2001).

In a data set that consisted of two national samples ($N = 7,774$), Mandl, Tronick, Brennan, Alpert, and Home (1999) found that several indicators of socioeconomic status were related to depression. Factors that predicted high levels of depression included age younger than twenty-one years, maternal level of education below high school, family income less than $20,000, Medicaid or self-pay insurance status, black race, and having given birth more than once.

Even among poor mothers, there is variation. In a study of 191 low-income women (Ritter et al. 2000), women with a higher relative income, who had social support and higher self-esteem, had lower levels of depression. In another low-income minority sample, Yonkers et al. (2001) found that 37 percent had depressive symptoms, and 6.5 to 8.5 percent met criteria for major depression. The authors did not support the hypothesis that postpartum major depression was more common in this population, however.

International Studies

Low socioeconomic status is a risk factor for depression in other countries as well. Patel et al. (2001) noted that depression is common in developing countries, and a vicious cycle of poverty, depression, and disability often occurs. This is especially true for women. In a sample from India, economic deprivation and a poor marital relationship were both important risk factors in the development of postpartum depression and in its continuing past six months postpartum (Patel et al., 2002). Other poverty-related variables, such as hunger and low education, were also associated with depression. This entire sample had low income. Even so, relative poverty made a difference. Similarly, in a sample of 257 Turkish women, living in a shanty was one predictor of depression (Danaci et al., 2002).

Boyce and colleagues (1998) had similar findings in their sample of 193 low-income mothers of school-age children. This sample was recruited from housing projects in Australia. The rate of current major depression was 17 percent, and the lifetime incidence of major depression was 29 percent. The depressed women in this sample reported low parental care during their childhoods and lack of current partner support. The depressed women also were more likely to have a vulnerable personality style, more stressful life events, and a lack of social support.

In an Irish sample from a disadvantaged neighborhood, 28 percent of 377 women were depressed when contacted a year after birth. The four risk factors associated with their depression were lower age, lack of a confidant, previous miscarriage, and previous treatment for depression (Cryan et al., 2001).

In a South African sample of poor women at two months post-partum, Cooper et al. (1999) found that an astonishing 35 percent met criteria for major depression. The authors found that depression was associated with poor partner support and an unplanned pregnancy: 69 percent of depressed mothers reported that their pregnancy had been unplanned.

Watson and Evans (1986) assessed three groups of new mothers in Great Britain: indigenous (English), Bengali, and "other" immigrants, including West Indians, Vietnamese, Chinese, Egyptians, and Sikhs. The results of their study indicated that while depression appeared in all three groups, the problems continued past the first postpartum year for the poorer groups. The authors suggested that the risk of continuing depression is greater when women have ongoing problems.

Debt is one aspect of poverty that has been specifically related to depression. In a longitudinal study of 271 families with young children, worry about debt was the strongest predictor of depression in mothers at the initial and follow-up contacts (Reading & Reynolds, 2001). Indeed, worrying about debt predicted depression six months later. Other economic factors associated with depression included overall family income, not being a homeowner, and lack of access to a car.

Although poverty is a risk factor, and depression occurs in low-income communities, we should not assume that all low-income populations have higher levels of depression. Indeed, as I describe in subsequent sections, some populations with much lower incomes are doing some very important things in terms of protecting new mothers. And even within a low-income population, higher relative income, social support, and high self-esteem buffer the effects of poverty.

MATERNITY LEAVE AND EMPLOYMENT

Maternity leave and decision making about returning to work can also influence depression. In one study, 570 pregnant women were interviewed at five months gestation and at one and four months postpartum (Hyde, Klein, Essex, & Clark, 1995). At the four-month interview, there was no difference in depression or anger based on return to work. But full-time workers had more anxiety. Women who took the shortest leaves (less than six weeks) and were high on marital concerns had the highest depression scores. The authors concluded that short maternity leaves, especially when combined with other risk factors, increased the risk for depression in new mothers.

Similarly, 436 women completed questionnaires five times during the postpartum period: at one month, three months, six months, nine months, and twelve months (Gjerdingen & Chaloner, 1994). Women had the highest levels of depression and anxiety at one month and the lowest levels at twelve months. Employment had a significant impact on depression, especially longer work hours and a maternity leave of less than twenty-four weeks. Other factors, such as maternal fatigue, loss of sleep, concern about appearance, and infant illness were also related to depression. Physical illness, previous mental illness, poor social support, fewer recreational activities, young age, and low income all contributed to depression as well.

Another study interviewed mothers three weeks before they started full-time out-of-home care for their babies and followed them over the next six months. Employed mothers who were working but wanted to be home were more depressed than mothers who were working and wanted to work. The children of mothers who wanted to be home but were working were also more likely to experience unstable care. Early entry into care was related to higher income, less maternal depression, and the use of family home care (McKim, Cramer, Stuart, & O'Connor, 1999).

A Canadian study of 447 mothers examined the relationship between employment status and depressive symptoms at six months postpartum (Des Rivieres-Pigeon, Seguin, Goulet, & Descarries, 2001). The authors found that women on maternity leave or women who were employed had the lowest levels of depression. Women at home full-time were more likely to report a lack of social support and to have an unwanted or mistimed pregnancy.

From these studies, it appears that women who have good support and have control over when (or if) they return to work have the lowest levels of depression. But other psychosocial variables, such as previous depression and lack of social support, continue to have an influence, in addition to maternity leave and employment.

SOCIAL SUPPORT

This was the first grandchild on my side. I thought everyone would come to see me. My mom did, but only after I called and asked her to come. My dad came the next day, but only for the day. . . . I was very isolated after the baby. I had no friends with babies. It was hard. . . . I thought my family would come and everyone would hold the baby. Everyone came to my house at Christmas and they spent six hours in the basement playing video games. I was really hurt by that. Nobody would help me. I've really never said anything. Maybe it would have been better if I had said something. (DeeDee)

Of the social factors considered, far and away the most influential is a woman's level of social support. As the research on nonpostpartum depression has repeatedly demonstrated, lack of social support is related to depression. This is especially true when women are faced with stressful life events. Social support is also related to many of the factors described in the previous chapters. It increases self-esteem and self-efficacy, acts as a buffer when a woman is faced with a temperamentally difficult child, and can even alter a woman's attributional style. Therefore, it becomes apparent that any effort to prevent postpartum depression must include a strong component of social support. The social support literature has included general support, partner support, and the impact of the social network. These studies are described next.

General Support

In a study of 191 low-income women, Ritter et al. (2000) found that women with good social support were less likely to become depressed. Social support was also significantly related to self-esteem; women who had high levels of support were also more likely to have high levels of self-esteem. Similarly, a Chinese study found that women with less social support were significantly more likely to become depressed (Xu & Lu, 2001).

In a prospective hospital-based study, Webster, Linnane, Dibley, and Pritchard (2000) found that low social support was strongly related to depression at sixteen weeks postpartum. Several types of support were specifically related to depression, including low support from friends, low family support, conflict with partner, and feeling unloved by partner. Also, 51 percent of the depressed women had a score of 25 or below on the Maternity Social Support Scale, while only 32 percent of the nondepressed women had this score.

In another study, Webster, Linnane, Dibley, Hinson, et al. (2000) found that social support was related to physical health and depression. Women with low support during pregnancy were more likely to report poorer health during pregnancy and after delivery. They were more likely to delay seeking prenatal care but to seek medical care more frequently once they did. They were more likely to be depressed in the postpartum period. Webster et al. found that women under age twenty were most likely to be in the low-support group, but overall the ages were comparable for low, medium, and adequate support.

In Cutrona's (1984) study of seventy-one primiparous women, overall level of support predicted depression in the later weeks of the postpartum period. The two aspects of social support that were most predictive of depression were *social integration* (the network of people with whom the mother shares interests and concerns) and *reliable alliance* (people whom the mother can count on for help in any circumstance). Cutrona explained her findings about the linkages of social support to postpartum depression by noting that contact with others may have helped the woman solve problems, led to her developing less threatening attributions about problems, provided opportunities for reinforcement from others, and increased her self-esteem and self-efficacy beliefs.

Social support provided by professionals (social workers) and nonprofessionals (experienced mothers) significantly lowered levels of anxiety in highly anxious primiparous women (Barnett & Parker, 1985). In addition, social support can benefit the mother-child relationship by helping mothers be more sensitive to their infants in the first year (Crockenberg & McCluskey, 1986). This trend continued until the children were older. In a study of thirty-eight mother-child dyads (with children ages twenty-seven to fifty-five months), the more support a mother received, the better were her interactions with her child. This result applied to single mothers and those in two-parent families (Weinraub & Wolf, 1987). In general, mothers with high support are more satisfied with their babies, their maternal roles, and their lives overall (Crnic & Greenberg, 1987).

Support from mothers' and fathers' own parents is also important (Matthey, Barnett, Ungerer, & Waters, 2000). In an Australian sample of 157 couples, relationships with their own mothers and fathers were important for both men and women. However, the best predictors of maternal and paternal mood at all time points were antenatal mood and relationship with partner.

Partner Support

Husbands or partners are also a key source of social support. Several studies have found that when that partner support is not available, mothers are more likely to be depressed. O'Hara (1986) found that depressed women reported less instrumental and emotional support from their husbands than did their nondepressed counterparts. In a prospective study of 730 women, depressed women reported lower marital satisfaction than nondepressed women (Gotlib et al., 1991). Similarly, low marital satisfaction and low overall ratings of the marriage were related to higher levels of postpartum depression (Watson et al., 1984). Depressed women were more likely to report that their marriage deteriorated postpartum than their nondepressed counterparts (Cox, Connor, & Kendell, 1982). In Turkey, women who had poor relationships with their spouses or their in-laws were at increased risk for depression in the first six months postpartum (Danaci et al., 2002). In her meta-analysis, Beck (2001) found quality of the marital relationship had a small effect size relative to postpartum depression.

The spouse's amount of help with child care and household tasks predicted depression severity at two months postpartum in another study (Campbell et al., 1992). Furthermore, spousal support interacted with pregnancy and delivery complications so that women with more complications and lower levels of support were more likely to be severely depressed. In this same study, women with less spousal support were also more likely to be chronically depressed, even up to two years later.

Another study attempted to determine the importance of social support with three samples of postpartum women: 105 middle-class white women, 37 middle-class mothers of premature babies, and 57 low-income African-American mothers (Logsdon & Usui, 2001). The authors tested a causal model, using structural equation modeling, and found that importance of support, support received, and closeness to partner were all significant predictors of both self-esteem and depression. These predictors were the same for all three groups of mothers.

In comparing 193 mothers and fathers on levels of postpartum depression, Dudley, Roy, Kelk, and Bernard (2001) found that fathers may be even more influenced by the quality of the relationship than mothers. Mothers' depression was influenced primarily by their own personalities (especially neuroticism), and perinatal and infant-related factors. In contrast, fathers were more influenced by the mothers' personality difficulties, unresolved past events, the mothers' current mental health, infant difficulties, and the state of their relationship. Depression in one partner was moderately correlated with depression in the other.

A study of 107 husbands and wives after the birth of their first child had similar findings. Lutz and Hock (2002) found that men who were less satisfied with their marriages were more likely to be depressed. For both men and women, fear of abandonment and fear of loneliness were significantly related to depressive symptoms. These relationships were stronger for men than for women in the sample.

Lack of support from fathers predicted the attribution style of high illusory control (Donovan & Leavitt, 1989), and perceived lack of support from fathers was also related to insecure attachments between thirty-four Japanese mothers and their twelve-month-old infants (Durrett, Otaki, & Richards, 1984). The authors concluded that mothers who did not have support might have higher levels of stress, making them psychologically unavailable to their infants.

Partner support also proved helpful in treatment of postpartum depression. In a sample of twenty-nine women with postpartum depression, thirteen were randomly assigned to receive psychoeducation for seven sessions. The second group had partners participate in four of the seven sessions. At the conclusion of the study, women whose partners were included in the intervention had significantly decreased depressive symptoms compared with the women whose partners were not included (Misri, Kostaras, Fox, & Kostaras, 2000).

These studies demonstrate that partner support can be a key factor in overcoming depression. It can also be helpful to include partners in interventions, especially because they may be affected by postpartum events and may also be depressed.

Social Network

Another aspect of social support research involves the entire social network. Certain features of the network that are of interest to researchers include the total size of the network (number of people it involves), number of confidants, proportion of kin, frequency of contact, and reciprocity in supportive interactions. O'Hara, Rehm, and Campbell (1983) examined these factors related to social networks, comparing a sample of depressed ($N = 11$) and nondepressed ($N = 19$) puerperal women. They found no significant difference in size of the social network and number of confidants for the two groups. Also, proportion of kin in the social network was not significantly different. But depressed subjects actually had more contact with their network than did their nondepressed counterparts. In spite of this increased level of contact, depressed women reported receiving less emotional and instrumental support. The major differences between the groups appeared to be in the abilities of each at giving and receiving support. The depressed women reported that they gave less support to their spouses, parents, and confidants, and received less emotional support from this same group. The authors hypothesized that this lower level of social support is an effect rather than a cause of the depression in that depressed people often become aversive to family and friends. In addition, friends or family may be uncomfortable dealing with someone who is depressed and may limit or avoid contact. Joanne describes this reaction from most of her friends, but noted that one friend continued to reach out to her.

I was usually an outgoing person, but I didn't have the energy to relate to others. My friends didn't know what to do. They thought I had had a nervous breakdown. Many stayed away. Even now, many are surprised that I can still function. I had one friend who was very supportive and loving continually, even though she didn't understand. She brought meals, wrote little notes. She made no demands on my recovery. My mother-in-law and husband were helpful during that time too.

The relationship between social support and depression appears to be bidirectional. Lack of social support increases the likelihood of depression, and depression seems to impair people's abilities to make social connections. A study (Hammen & Brennan, 2002) sought to explore this relationship in a community sample of 812 women. They were divided into three groups: formerly depressed, currently depressed, and never depressed. Data were collected from spouses, adolescent children, and independent raters. Their findings demonstrated that interpersonal difficulties are not simply consequences of depressive symptoms. Women who were not currently depressed, but formerly had been, were more impaired on every measure of interpersonal behavior and beliefs than women who were never depressed. There were many indices of problems. Their marriages were less stable. They had poorer marital satisfaction. More spousal coercion and injury occurred. They had more problems in their relationships with their children, friends, and extended families. Their lives were more stressful, and they experienced more stressful life events. Finally, they were more insecure in their beliefs about others. The authors concluded that interpersonal difficulties were a stable component of depression and that these difficulties were not only difficult to treat but could make sufferers more vulnerable to future episodes of depression.

Why Social Support Is Sometimes Stressful

As the previously cited studies demonstrate, social support is important for mental health. But sometimes "support" may not be helpful. When considering whether a woman is receiving adequate support, it is easy to be fooled by appearances. We might assume that a woman who knows a lot of people, or is receiving assistance, is experiencing social support. But this is not always the case. People in a woman's social network might not offer to help. Even if they do help, the woman must perceive it as support. Unwanted help can undermine a woman's confidence in her mothering abilities, threaten her self-esteem, and engender dependency on the person providing the help. Even when a woman is grateful for the assistance, she may be uncomfortable accepting it if she is an independent or private person and is used to doing things for herself (Affleck et al., 1989). Christine describes how having her mother and her in-laws come to help after the baby was born made her uncomfortable.

Everyone was really helping with the baby but me. They were *too* supportive. I know my husband wouldn't want to think that. I felt like they were taking over everything, that I had to be able to do it all. I kept trying to be the perfect wife. I'm a very private person. I felt like everything was exposed.

People who are overburdened and overstressed may withdraw from others so that they do not have to provide support. Unfortunately, people who are depressed are often the ones who most need help from others and are least likely to get it. To examine this issue, Riley and Eckenrode (1986) randomly selected 356 low-income women from a neighborhood health clinic in Boston. They measured social support and personal resources, which consisted of financial and psychological resources related to effective coping. As predicted, social support actually increased negative affect for women with low resources. These women were at much higher risk from the "contagion of stress" phenomenon. "The low-resource women, when faced with many stressful events happening to others, are more distressed because they are less able to give the material and emotional support expected of them" (p. 777). They concluded that a large social network was beneficial for high-resource women, but was actually harmful for low-resource women.

A similar pattern was found in families who were maltreating their children. Gaudin, Polansky, Kilpatrick, and Shilton (1993) compared neglectful low-income mothers with those who were low-income but not neglectful. There were striking differences between the groups. The neglectful mothers were significantly lonelier and more socially isolated, they reported more depression, and averaged more than twice the number of stressful life events in the previous year. They reported fewer social ties, and more people in their social networks were critical of them. It is unlikely that neglect causes loneliness, although some parents may be rejected because of their lifestyles. However, loneliness might lead to despondency that could lead to neglect. The authors recommended that case workers address loneliness and isolation in these families to help them cope with significant life stresses related to poverty and lack of access to health care, housing, and other support services.

A study comparing 670 nonabusing families with 166 abusive families found similar results (Gracia & Musitu, 2003). The families in this sample were Colombian and Spanish. The authors found that in both cultures, abusive parents showed lower levels of community integration, participation in social activities, and use of formal and informal organizations than parents who were providing adequate care for their children. The abusive parents tended to be more socially isolated and negative in their attitudes toward their community and neighborhood.

The Role of Culture: Social Structures That Protect New Mothers

The studies just cited focus on women's networks involving family or friends; how they are helpful and how they may lead to even more stress. Another type of research on social support has examined the role of the culture in which women live. Stern and Kruckman (1983), in their classic article, found that depression, or even the postpartum blues, are virtually nonexistent in several cultures around the world. Although these cultures differed dramatically from one another, they had common elements. The characteristics of this type of support are listed in the following sections.

A Distinct Postpartum Period

In almost all the societies studied, the postpartum period was recognized as a time that is distinct from normal life. Postpartum is a time when mothers are supposed to recuperate, their activities are limited, and they are taken care of by female relatives. This was also common practice in colonial America and was referred to as the "lying-in" period (Wertz & Wertz, 1989).

Protective Measures Reflecting the New Mother's Vulnerability

During the postpartum period, new mothers are recognized as being especially vulnerable. In some cultures, the postpartum period is considered a time of ritual uncleanness, while in others it is a time for mothers to rest, regain strength, and care for their babies. Many rituals are associated with vulnerability, such as the eating or avoidance of certain foods, wrapping of mother's head or abdomen, and limitations on the amount of company she receives. All of these rituals protect the mother and set aside the postpartum period as distinct from normal life.

Social Seclusion and Mandated Rest

Related to the concept of vulnerability is the widespread practice of social seclusion for new mothers. During this time, she is supposed to rest and restrict normal activities. In the Punjab, women are secluded from everyone but female relatives and the midwife for five days. After the five days, there is a "stepping out" ceremony for the mother and baby. In other cultures, the time of seclusion can be as long as three months. Seclusion and rest also allow mothers to recover, promote breastfeeding, and limits their normal activities.

Functional Assistance

To make sure that women get the rest they need, they must be relieved of their normal workload. Functional assistance involves care of older children, household help, and personal attendance during labor. As in the colonial period in the United States, women often return to their family homes to ensure that this type of assistance is available.

Social Recognition of a Mother's New Role and Status

In cultures with a low incidence of the blues or depression, a great deal of personal attention is given to the mother. This has been described as "mothering the mother." In these various cultures, the new status of the mother is recognized through social rituals and gifts. For example, in Punjabi culture, the mother receives the ritual stepping-out ceremony, ritual bathing and hair washing performed by the midwife, and a ceremonial meal prepared by a Brahman. When she returns to her husband's family, she returns with many gifts she has been given for herself and the baby. Ritual bathing, washing of hair, massage, binding of the abdomen, and other types of personal care are also prominent in the postpartum rituals of rural Guatemala, among Mayan women in the Yucatan, and among Latina women in both the United States and Mexico. Here is a description of a recognition ritual performed by the Chagga people of Uganda:

> Three months after the birth of her child, the Chagga woman's head is shaved and crowned with a bead tiara, she is robed in an ancient skin garment worked with beads, a staff such as the el-

ders carry is put in her hand, and she emerges from her hut for her first public appearance with her baby. Proceeding slowly towards the market, they are greeted with songs such as are sung to warriors returning from battle. She and her baby have survived the weeks of danger. The child is no longer vulnerable, but a baby who has learned what love means, has smiled its first smiles, and is now ready to learn about the bright, loud world outside. (Dunham, 1992, p. 148)

Even in the absence of these type of rituals, mothers need physical nurturance. Professional postpartum doula Salle Webber describes what mothers need in the first few weeks after birth:

> In my work as a Doula, my focus is on the mother. . . . A mother needs someone who cares about how many times the baby woke to nurse in the night, how many diapers were changed, how her breasts are feeling. She may need her back massaged or her sheets changed, or she may need someone to provide an abundant supply of water or tea, salads ready-made in the refrigerator, a bowl of cut-up fruit. . . . She may have many questions and concerns that only an experienced mother can understand. She needs patience and kind words and a clean and calm environment. (Webber, 1992, p. 17)

What Mothers Usually Face

These forms of protection and help are a far cry from what mothers in the United States and other industrialized nations often receive postpartum. After a baby is born in mainstream U.S. culture, all the attention shifts from the mother to the baby. One popular book written for new mothers (Eisenberg, Murkoff, & Hathaway, 1989) describes this transition as "the reverse Cinderella—the pregnant princess has become the postpartum peasant" with a "wave of the obstetrician's wand" (p. 546). Many of the mothers interviewed for this book felt a profound sense of loss and abandonment by their medical caregivers and their families. In general, they received little acknowledgment of what they had been through, both physically and emotionally, by giving birth.

I really wanted someone to make me feel special. All the attention was on the baby. (Barbara)

I feel a sense of anticlimax. I was used to being the center of attention. Then I had to go back to being a normal healthy person. I'm not begging for attention, but now everyone only pays attention to the baby. It would be nice to have some attention afterward. While you're pregnant, you're feeling fat and slobby, and don't want it. After the baby, you want it. (Julie)

I felt like I didn't matter. I felt like they weren't interested in me after I had my baby. . . . My husband said, "of course they are not interested. You've had your baby." The six-week visit seemed like an eternity away. I wrote [my midwife] a note to thank her. She didn't even mention it when I saw her at six weeks. . . . When I felt great, they treated me nicely. Now when I feel so awful with this baby, no one seems to be available to me. (Karen)

My doctor thought her job was done after my daughter was born. It's ridiculous to think the job is done just because you've delivered the baby. I called her a couple of times after, and she told me to see a social worker. I eventually left my OB. There were many reasons, but mainly because she left me high and dry after delivery. (Jan)

After the birth, I had several people tell me that the most important thing was that I had a healthy baby. Yes, that is important. But what about me? No one pays attention to the fact that you've had major surgery. They would have paid more attention if you had had your appendix out. (Sally)

Rothman (1982), in her sociological analysis of American childbirth practices, describes how pregnancy, childbirth, and the postpartum period are often viewed as discrete events instead of different stages of the same process. This could account for some of the profound letdown that many women feel. Oakley (1983) points out that normal care of a newborn involves many activities that would be forbidden for days or even weeks following abdominal surgery, but are expected of women following cesarean section. In the United States in particular, the lying-in period tends to end when the woman leaves the hospital (O'Hara, 1986). These authors stated that a key to prevention of postpartum depression lies in continuation of the caregiving process through the end of the postpartum period and beyond.

Are All Rituals Helpful?

Stern and Kruckman (1983) present these structural differences in cultures as evidence indicating that the high incidence of postpartum mental illness in the United States and other industrialized nations is "culture bound." Cox (1988), however, pointed out that it is naive and inaccurate to claim that postpartum illness does not occur in non-Western cultures. As I described in Chapter 1, postpartum mental illness occurs in countries all over the world. Cox's research in East Africa also found elaborate social rituals associated with delivery and a high incidence of both postpartum depression and psychosis. He concluded that postpartum illness cannot be considered merely a cultural artifact.

The differences in the two analyses may be found in the definition of social rituals. In Stern and Kruckman (1983), social rituals provided support to the mother. She was given personal attention and care, and temporarily relieved of her day-to-day duties. The rituals described by Cox (1988) focused on the legitimacy of the baby. For example, an older woman was assigned to the pregnant woman to be sure that no taboos were violated that could call into question the legitimacy of her child (such as not allowing a man to step over her legs). Another ritual was that her husband's clan, to ensure legitimacy of her child, examined a naked pregnant woman. After birth, the midwife determined legitimacy by seeing if the umbilical cord floated when put in a mixture of beer, milk, and water. Any difficulties a mother encountered during labor were said to be a result of her own immorality. These rituals acted as tests of legitimacy and were not supportive toward a mother. In fact, they probably increased her stress level. (The author does not state what happened to babies who were determined to be illegitimate, but it is probably not good.)

It is safe to conclude that the existence of rituals is not enough to ensure that women do not suffer from postpartum illness. The type of rituals is also important. Rituals that appear to be effective in preventing postpartum illness are those that provide support and assistance for new mothers.

Summary

Social factors have a significant role to play in the development of postpartum depression. Women who experience stressful life events during the childbearing year are at increased risk for depression, as are mothers at both ends of the age continuum. Low income can also make mothers vulnerable to depression, but not in all cases. Social support can be an important buffer against life stress. But sometimes support is not perceived as helpful, and can actually make matters worse. Beyond a woman's immediate circle of family and friends, an entire culture can determine whether mothers are vulnerable to depression.

SUPPORTING THE MOTHER-INFANT RELATIONSHIP

Throughout this chapter, I have described the importance of relationships as a buffer against the stresses associated with the postpartum period. Summing up, another way to conceptualize all the risk factors from Chapters 3 to 7 is in terms of their impact on the mother-infant relationship. This conceptualization is also summarized in Table 7.1.

What Hinders the Relationship?

So in terms of what I have described in previous chapters, what types of things would hinder the mother/infant relationship? Fatigue certainly could. A mother who is exhausted is going to have little left to give to her baby. Postpartum pain can also keep the mother's focus away from her baby. A negative childbirth experience can leave mothers feeling very disconnected from or even angry with their babies. Mothers who feel incompetent or bad about themselves as mothers may avoid taking care of their babies. Mothers who have a history of abuse or neglect, and who have never dealt with it, may have difficulties when they become mothers. A crying baby can certainly push a mother over the edge and may make her feel very angry. Similarly, a baby who is having breastfeeding difficulties, especially one that actively refuses the breast, may be difficult for the mother. Finally, mothers with little support may find themselves so overwhelmed that they cannot cope with the demands of motherhood.

TABLE 7.1. Supporting the mother-infant relationship.

Supports the mother-infant relationship	Can hinder the mother-infant relationship
• Adequate rest and nutrition • Positive or resolved birth experience • Accurate and timely information • Emotional support • Practical assistance • Respite from infant care • Maternal self-efficacy/self-esteem • Realistic expectations of self and infant • Understanding of temperament • Positive breastfeeding experience	• Fatigue • Postpartum pain • Negative or traumatic childbirth experience • Unrealistic expectations of self or infant • Low self-esteem/self-efficacy • Unresolved history of abuse or family dysfunction • Infant's difficult temperament • Infant health issues • Breastfeeding difficulties • Lack of social support • Overwhelming child care responsibiities

What Supports the Relationship?

Conversely, what elements support the mother-infant relationship? For starters, a mother who receives adequate rest and good nutrition will be able to give more easily to others, including her new baby. A mother with a positive or resolved birth experience will be free to connect with her baby. Accurate and timely information can make a difference for a mother who is struggling. Emotional support and practical assistance can also make her transition easier and can allow her to focus on the baby. Occasional respite from infant care, even thirty minutes to take a shower, can help her return to her baby more focused, knowing that her own needs have been met. Mothers who feel competent and who have realistic expectations of themselves and their babies are going to enjoy the experience of mothering more than someone who always feels that she is not living up to what she "should" be doing. Along the same line, a realistic perspective on temperament can help mothers not blame themselves for their infants' behaviors. Finally, a positive breastfeeding experience can help mothers experience the joys of mothering, knowing that they are giving their babies something no one else can.

If we focus on helping mothers have a positive relationship with their babies, many of the other difficulties will fall by the wayside. In the next four chapters, I describe assessment of postpartum depression and the wide range of treatment options.

Chapter 8

Assessment of Postpartum Depression

Over the past fifteen years, researchers have repeatedly demonstrated that postpartum depression is quite treatable. These treatment options are described in Chapters 9 through 11. But before depression can be treated, it must be identified. This chapter describes some techniques and instruments for screening for depression in health care and other settings.

CHALLENGES TO ASSESSING POSTPARTUM DEPRESSION

Beck (1993) described postpartum depression as a thief that robs women of happiness during their first weeks and months as mothers. It is stealth; as many as 50 percent of cases are not identified (Beck & Gable, 2001b; Cooper & Murray, 1998). In a study of 1,102 new mothers (MacLennan, Wilson, & Taylor, 1996), only 49 percent of women with serious depression sought help for it. In another study, health care providers did not identify almost half of the depressed mothers. These mothers made an average of fourteen health care visits each (Hearn et al., 1998). Mothers themselves contribute to this dismal record in that they often go to great lengths to conceal their depression from health care providers, as well as friends and family (Beck & Gable, 2001b). But health care providers also fail to identify depression, even when mothers see them on a regular basis (Cooper & Murray, 1998).

Use of Health Care Services

One clue that depressed mothers provide is increased use of health care services. In an Australian study (Webster et al., 2001), depressed mothers made more visits to the pediatrician or their primary care provider. They were also significantly more likely to visit a psychiatrist or social worker, to seek the assistance of a postpartum depression support group, and to contact the Nursing Mothers' Association of Australia. Also, they were significantly less satisfied with those services. The women were unhappy because they felt that their providers did not listen and because of the poor quality of information they received. Webster et al. speculated that the mothers could be unhappy because the real reason for their visit (i.e., depression) was not identified. They also found that women rarely raised the issue of depression themselves, but provided hints to their providers about the way they were feeling. The authors recommended the use of screening questions to help mothers raise these issues when consulting with health care providers.

Another large study of women at three to eight weeks postpartum (N = 7,794) also found that health care use predicted depression. Mothers were significantly more likely to be depressed if their infants had more than one problem-oriented visit to the infant's primary care provider, or if they made even one visit to the emergency department. The number of problem-oriented visits in the first month was positively associated with increased rates of depressive symptoms. This was also true in months two through five, but the relationship was weaker. Well-child visits were not associated with maternal depression (Mandl et al., 1999). The authors speculated on possible reasons for their findings. They felt that depression might color a mother's perceptions of the wellness of her infant. Mothers may also seek care for their infant as an indirect way to get care for themselves. Seeing a primary care provider may seem less stigmatizing than seeking help for depression. Conversely, mothers may be depressed because their infants are actually ill. We must be careful not to attribute all of a mother's concerns to depression.

Increased use of health care services comes at a substantial cost. In the Ontario Mother and Infant Survey (Roberts et al., 2001), mothers who were depressed and mothers who made less than $20,000 per year had the highest health care costs. The total health and social service costs were almost double for both groups (calculated separately) compared to the rest of the sample. Other variables that predicted higher health care costs included mothers' perception of their own health as poor, perception of inadequate help and support at home, and a postpartum hospital stay of less than forty-eight hours.

SCREENING FOR DEPRESSION

As indicated, women may provide clues that could indicate that they are depressed. Pay particular attention when women say they feel overwhelmed, that nothing will ever be the same, or that they feel hopeless or out of control. Also be alert when women describe anxiety, nervousness, or insomnia—especially early morning waking.

Morris-Rush and Bernstein (2002) indicated that screening for depression during the postpartum visit should be the standard of care, and that the health care setting is often a good place to screen. A study from a midwifery practice revealed a number of positive results from even the most rudimentary screening (Webster et al., 1997). In this study, women were asked about risk factors for postpartum depression while they were still pregnant. Women with risk factors were asked to complete the Edinburgh Postnatal Depression Scale (EPDS), and were then offered information about postpartum depression. A qualitative study was undertaken to evaluate the effectiveness of this intervention. The women who completed the EPDS were asked about their level of comfort in answering these questions. The majority felt comfortable and felt that the amount of information provided was appropriate. The hospital staff and midwives also found the intervention to be helpful. After the intervention, midwives and staff were much more likely to think that postpartum depression was within their realm of responsibility and were less likely to consider it a private matter.

The efficacy of screening by risk factors was demonstrated in another study by the same authors (Webster, Linnane, Dibley, & Pritchard, 2000). In this study, 2,118 women were screened during pregnancy. Of these women, 691 (32.6 percent) had one or more risk factors for depression. The women were then contacted at four months postpartum and asked to complete the EPDS. Of women with one or more risk factors, 26 percent scored above 12 (the cutoff for depression), compared with only 11 percent of the women who did not have any risk factors prenatally. The risk of depression increased with the number of risk factors. Forty-eight percent of the women with five risk factors had EPDS scores above 12. The authors felt they could have improved predictions by adding questions about infant behavior, severe blues, and childhood abuse. They acknowledged that many of the women in their local postpartum support group were sexual abuse survivors, and adding this variable would have improved detection rates. Nevertheless, even without this variable, they found that it was useful to screen for risk factors in the antenatal clinic.

In a study of family physicians, Worrall, Angel, Chaulk, Clarke, and Robbins (1999) found only a modest improvement in the identification and treatment of patients with depression in a general practice. The physicians in the intervention group participated in a three-hour training session on clinical practice guidelines for depression. After the intervention, physicians in the intervention group identified more depression and referred more patients to psychiatrists and other mental health professionals. But this number was not significantly different than physicians in the control group. Nevertheless, it was an improvement and indicates that training can be helpful.

General Questions to Screen for Depressive Symptoms

Patients may have symptoms of depression without meeting criteria for major depression. To identify these women, you may have to ask specific questions. General questions such as, "how's everything going?" are likely to elicit responses such as "fine," with no further elaboration about their distress. Examples of more effective questions are: "Have you been feeling sad?" "Have you been crying lately?" "How much?" "Do you feel you are a good mother?" "Are you enjoying the baby?" Sometimes even asking these types of questions can validate a woman's feelings and give her permission to tell you how she really feels.

Following are some additional general questions that can be used as an initial screen for depression. Patients who are having difficulty with one or more of these questions may need further screening. Most mothers may answer "yes" to both fatigue questions from this series. But mothers who seem more fatigued than other mothers may be depressed and merit further screening (Institute for Clinical Systems Improvement, 2000).

Have you had any difficulty sleeping?
Have you been more tired or less active than usual?
Have you felt more stressed than usual?
Have you been less interested in interacting with others, including your partner, friends, or children?

ASSESSMENT SCALES

Beyond these general questions, a screening scale is often helpful. Fortunately, there are two screening scales designed specifically for postpartum women. These are described next.

The Edinburgh Postnatal Depression Scale

One of the most commonly used screening and diagnostic tools for postpartum depression is the EPDS, a ten-item self-report questionnaire that can be completed in five minutes (Cox, Holden, & Sagovsky, 1987). It was designed to give primary care providers and other health care workers a simple tool for screening in the postpartum period. Women are asked to report how they have felt in the past week, and the items are scored from 0 to 3. A score greater than 12 indicates possible depression. It has been used in numerous research studies, in populations all over the world, and it is available free of charge. (A downloadable version of the EPDS is available at <www.GraniteScientific.com>. The authors have granted the right to use their questionnaire without charge or permission as long as the source of the scale is listed and the copyright is respected.) Since it has been used in so many different countries, O'Hara (1994) argues that it could be used epidemiologically for comparing rates of postpartum depression across cultures.

The EPDS offers a number of advantages. It is easy to complete and score. Mothers can answer all the questions in a few minutes. It is specifically written for new mothers. Indeed, it was because of the limitations of the more generic depression measures that the EPDS was developed. O'Hara (1994) reviewed some of the problems with other measures of depression that are used in postpartum depression research. The first is the Beck Depression Inventory (BDI), written by Aaron Beck. This is a twenty-one-item self-report inventory that can be used in the general population. One limitation is that some of the symptoms on this scale could be true for most new mothers, not just those who are depressed. For example, O'Hara pointed out that seven of the items on the BDI are concerned with somatic symptoms. These somatic symptoms are a normal part of the postpartum experience (e.g., changes in appetite, sleep, energy). The Zung Self-Rating Depression Scale, although used less frequently, has a number of problems similar to the BDI, particularly the emphasis on somatic symptoms, and can yield false positives.

Although widely used, the EPDS has some disadvantages. The scale is written in British rather than American English. American mothers may find the wording of some the questions confusing or a little odd. Lappin (2001) cautions that the EPDS is designed to be used in the early postpartum period and has only been validated for that use. It should not be used for screening for depression in pregnancy or to diagnose depression beyond the postpartum period. But it is often used in both of these situations. Lappin (2001) also cautions against interpreting one- or two-point differences as indicating increased severity. This instrument does its best predicting depression with a cutoff of twelve points. Similarly, Elliot and Leverton (2000) noted that the EPDS is a reliable and valid screening tool, but it has been misused. They emphasized the importance of ongoing training and quality control to ensure that it is used properly.

Another caution comes from Guedeney, Fermanian, Guelfi, and Kumar (2000). They provided a case report of three false negatives on the EPDS with women with major depressive disorder (according to another measure of depression, the Research Diagnostic Criteria). They noted that the EPDS seems better able to identify depressed postpartum women with anhedonic and anxious symptoms than depressed women with psychomotor retardation.

Despite these limitations, it is a useful tool. A wide range of studies have used the EPDS and compared its scores with those of other depression assessment tools. These studies are summarized in Table 8.1.

TABLE 8.1. Studies using the Edinburgh Postnatal Depression Scale (EPDS).

Study population	Authors	Conclusions
48 Bangladeshi women EPDS translated to Syhleti/Bengali	Fuggle, Glover, Khan & Haydon, 2002	The EDPS worked well with this sample. Some difficulty translating item 1. Compared results with the General Health Questionnaire.
88 Japanese mothers Assessed early post-partum disturbance	Yamashita, Yoshida, Nakano, & Tashiro, 2000	Compared EPDS to other instruments. EPDS identified all depressed mothers at 1 month postpartum.
892 women from 9 countries (U.S., Guyana, Italy, Sweden, Finland, Korea, Taiwan, India, and Australia)	Affonso et al., 2000	Moderate concordance between Beck Depression Inventory and EPDS. Authors concluded that both are useful for screening and assessment. Also useful with a diverse, international population.
100 Nepalese women, 2-3 months postpartum; 40 control women	Regmi et al., 2002	EPDS is a reliable and easy-to-use tool for PPD screening.
145 Chinese women at 6 weeks postpartum	Lee, Yip, Chiu, & Chung, 2000	Compared EPDS and General Health Questionnaire. Substantial improvement in screening when both instruments are used than when either form is used alone.
Low-income American sample Two conditions: 35 routine clinical evaluation, 37 using EPDS	Fergerson, Jamieson, & Lindsay, 2002	The EDPS was significantly better than routine evaluations for identifying depression. 30 percent in EPDS group identified as "at risk" for depression; 0 percent in the clinical assessment group.
208 fathers EPDS scores compared with Diagnostic Interview Schedule	Matthey, Barnett, Kavanagh, & Howie, 2001	Authors conclude that the EPDS is a reliable and valid measure of depression and anxiety in mothers, but should have a cutoff two points lower for fathers than for mothers.

TABLE 8.1 *(continued)*

Study population	Authors	Conclusions
134 women at 6 weeks postpartum; 199 women at 3 months postpartum (EPDS and Present State Examination)	Leverton & Elliott, 2000	With a cutoff of 12-13, EPDS sensitivity = 70 percent, specificity = 93 percent. With a cutoff of 9-10, sensitivity = 90 percent, specificity = 84 percent. Home visitor description of women as depressed or "fed up" at 6 weeks was a better predictor than EPDS.
56 Norwegian women at 6 weeks postpartum	Eberhard-Gran, Eskild, Tambs, Schei, & Opjordsmoen, 2001	Cutoff $\geq$ 10 identified all women with major depression. 100 percent sensitivity, 87 percent specificity, but wide confidence intervals. Authors concluded that EPDS is a valid screening instrument for postpartum depression.
224 low-income Canadian mothers, 22nd and 35th days postpartum	Des Rivieres-Pigeon et al., 2000	Used a confirmatory factor analysis. Good construct validity for EPDS. Cronbach α = .82.

The Postpartum Depression Screening Scale

Another tool designed specifically for new mothers is the Postpartum Depression Screening Scale (PDSS), developed by Cheryl Beck. The PDSS is a thirty-five-item Likert-scale self-report instrument. It measures functioning on seven dimensions: sleeping/eating disturbances, anxiety/insecurity, emotional lability, cognitive impairment, loss of self, guilt/shame, and contemplating harming oneself. It takes five to ten minutes to complete, and is available for a small fee from Western Psychological Services <www.wpspublish.com>.

Like the EPDS, the PDSS is useful for screening mothers for depression. In addition, the subscales can provide information for clinicians in treating mothers by highlighting specific areas of difficulty. In developing this scale, Beck and Gable (2000) attempted to address the limitations of the EPDS. For example, they noted that the EPDS did not measure postpartum feelings such as loss of control, loneliness, irritability, fear of going crazy, obsessive thinking, concentration difficulty, and loss of self. In a study of 525 new mothers, confirmatory factor analysis supported the seven dimensions of the PDSS. The internal consistencies on the seven dimensions ranged from 0.83 (sleeping/eating disturbances) to 0.94 (loss of self). A panel of experts also established the content validity of the scale, and item-response theory techniques provided further construct validity (Beck & Gable, 2000).

In another study (Beck & Gable, 2001a, 2001b), 150 mothers at twelve weeks postpartum completed the PDSS, EPDS, and the Beck Depression Inventory-II. Following completion of these questionnaires, each woman was interviewed by a nurse/psychotherapist using the Structural Clinical Interview for DSM-IV Axis I disorders. The results of the PDSS correlated with the EPDS ($r = 0.79$) and the Beck ($r = 0.81$). The authors then performed a hierarchical regression to ascertain the level of variance that the PDSS accounted for above and beyond the other two measures. The results indicated that the PDSS accounted for an additional 9 percent of the variance in the diagnosis of depression. A cutoff score of 80 for major depression has a sensitivity of 94 percent and a specificity of 98 percent. A cutoff of 60 can be used for both major and minor depression and has a sensitivity of 91 percent and a specificity of 72 percent. The PDSS was superior in this sample in identifying major depression partly because it included items on sleep, cognitive impairment, and anxiety (Beck & Gable, 2001a).

ADDITIONAL FACTORS

Once you have determined that a mother is depressed, you must make some additional judgments to help you guide her to the right level of help and support. These additional factors include the severity of the current episode and whether she is abusing substances, at risk for suicide, or requires hospitalization.

Severity of Current Episode

After determining whether a mother is depressed, the next item of business is to evaluate the severity of her depression. In attempting to evaluate severity of the current episode, there are three factors to consider: duration of symptoms, intensity of symptoms, and level of impairment. Symptoms must be present for two weeks for a diagnosis of major depression. In cases of severe depression, it has often gone on much longer. Intensity of the symptoms and level of impairment can also indicate whether aggressive treatment is warranted. If patients suddenly stop paying attention to personal grooming, cannot manage their households, or have days when they cannot get out of bed, the depressive episode is most likely severe.

Assessing Active Substance Abuse

Another consideration is whether patients are actively abusing alcohol or drugs. Substance abuse can be comorbid with depression or PTSD. Since active substance abuse complicates treatment for depression, if it is detected, patients should be referred to a substance-abuse treatment program. Following are some screening questions for possible substance abuse (Institute for Clinical Systems Improvement, 2004).

Do you feel you should drink or use drugs less often?
Has a friend or family member told you to drink or use drugs less often?
Do you feel guilty when you drink or use drugs?

If a patient says yes to two or more of these questions, make a referral to a substance abuse program for further evaluation.

Assessing Suicide Risk

Suicide risk is always an important consideration when working with depressed mothers. Although it is rare, the consequences are so serious that it is helpful to screen all mothers who are depressed. The Institute for Clinical Systems Improvement (2004) gives some specific signs that may indicate increased suicide risk in the following list. Even with these signs, it is still difficult to predict suicide. Be sure to document your assessment of suicide risk in your patient records.

1. Has made other suicide attempts
2. Thinks about suicide or has made specific suicide plans
3. Abuses substances or is addicted
4. Personality disorder or psychosis
5. Family member has committed suicide
6. Single marital status
7. Recent death of a loved one
8. Recent divorce or separation
9. Insomnia not related to baby care
10. Panic attacks or severe anxiety
11. Diminished concentration
12. Severe anhedonia or hopelessness

Even one of these risk factors present may call for a more specialized consultation. According to Remick (2002), detailed suicide plans, social isolation, previous suicide attempts, substance abuse, and a family history of suicide all increase risk. These patients should be closely monitored through frequent visits, residing with family or friends, or by being hospitalized. Contact your local suicide-prevention hotline for information about how best to proceed and for referrals to people who can help. Ignoring suicide risk can be lethal.

Assessing the Need for Psychiatric Hospitalization

Finally, hospitalization may be necessary when severe symptoms are present. Particularly troubling are signs that mothers plan to harm themselves or their babies. When making a decision about whether psychiatric hospitalization is necessary, there are a few considerations (Institute for Clinical Systems Improvement, 2000):

Does the patient have suicidal thoughts or plans?
Do you fear for the patient's safety?
Does the patient have plans to assault or kill another person, including the baby?
Is there psychotic thinking?
Has the patient lost the ability to care for himself or herself?

Hospitalization can be voluntary or involuntary. If at all possible, try to find a hospital where mothers are allowed to have their babies stay with them. Some hospitals have mother/baby units that are designed with the needs of postpartum women in mind. Failing that, try to find a situation in which mothers can see their babies frequently.

If mothers are hospitalized while still breastfeeding, also try to make arrangements to protect their milk supply. These mothers need access to a hospital-grade electric pump. A regular schedule of pumping can ensure that the milk supply is maintained, help mothers avoid problems associated with sudden weaning (e.g., breast infections), and also gives mothers a vision of life beyond the hospital.

CONCLUSION

Mothers are often not forthcoming about their depression. They may not even realize that they are depressed. But they often know that something is wrong, which may prompt them to seek health care often for themselves and for their babies.

You can screen for depression by using some general questions about their level of fatigue and stress. You can also use one of the two screening measures designed specifically for new mothers. Screening can also help you determine whether a mother is suicidal, needs to be hospitalized, or needs a referral for other assistance.

Once depression has been identified, mothers need to be treated. A wide range of treatments is available for depressed new mothers. Most of these alternatives are compatible with breastfeeding. The treatments are the subject of the next three chapters.

Chapter 9

Alternative and Complementary Therapies: Diet, Supplements, and Exercise

Alternative and complementary medicine is increasingly popular with the general public. Under this broad heading are many treatment modalities, some of which are effective for treating depression. In this chapter, I describe three modalities—diet, supplements, and exercise—that can be used alone or as adjuncts to standard treatments of antidepressants and therapy. Herbal antidepressants, another alternative therapy, are described in Chapter 11. With each modality I also provide information about what mothers can do for themselves to help with their depression.

These three treatment modalities have a minimal impact on breastfeeding. The term *minimal impact* is used rather than *no impact* because supplements or exercise can, at least theoretically, influence a mother's milk. However, these effects are generally not a problem for most mothers.

DIET

The first treatment modality I describe is diet—specifically, the mood-altering effects of carbohydrates. Carbohydrates increase levels of the neurotransmitter serotonin by influencing insulin secretion and the plasma-tryptophan ratio (Wurtman & Wurtman, 1995). Serotonin is involved in sleep, pain sensitivity, blood pressure regulation, and mood. People low in serotonin often overeat carbohydrates in an attempt to self-medicate and feel better. Researchers have also examined the carbohydrate-mood connection with other populations who have conditions related to low levels of serotonin, such as people under stress and women with premenstrual syndrome (PMS) or obsessive-compulsive disorder (OCD).

Carbohydrates, Premenstrual Syndrome, and Obsessive-Compulsive Disorder

Women with PMS tend to crave carbohydrates. In a study of women with premenstrual syndrome (Wurtman, Brzezinski, Wurtman, & Laferrere, 1989), the authors compared nineteen women with severe PMS and nine control women. All the women were inpatients during the study. Women with PMS had a significant increase in carbohydrate intake during the late luteal stage of their menstrual cycles. During this time, the rate of carbohydrate consumption increased 24 percent during meals and 43 percent from snacks. Protein intake did not rise, but fat intake did because it was a component in many of the foods the women craved. Carbohydrate-rich/protein-poor foods improved depression, tension, anger, confusion, sadness, and fatigue, and increased alertness and calmness among the PMS patients. No such change occurred during the follicular stage for these women, or at either stage for women who did not have PMS.

Sayegh et al. (1995) also found that carbohydrates were beneficial for controlling symptoms of PMS. In this study, twenty-four women with confirmed PMS were enrolled in a double-blind study to test a carbohydrate-rich beverage versus a low-carbohydrate beverage. The women participated through three menstrual cycles, during the late luteal phase. The carbohydrate drink significantly decreased self-reported depression and increased memory-word recognition. The placebo drink had no effect on either of these measures.

Researchers have also noted high levels of carbohydrate craving in patients with OCD (O'Rourke et al., 1994). This study compared the snacking and eating patterns of 170 patients with OCD and 920 controls. The subjects showed significant differences in the amount of carbohydrate snacks consumed, with patients with OCD consuming more. These patients also had a positive mood response to these snacks. The authors noted that OCD is another condition that responds well to sertonergic drugs, and therefore seems related to levels of serotonin.

Stress and Carbohydrates

Serotonin levels are also often low in people under stress. In one study, the authors investigated whether a carbohydrate-rich/protein-poor diet would prevent depression and deterioration of mood and performance better than a protein-rich/carbohydrate-poor diet (Markus et al., 1998). This study operated under the assumption that stress depletes serotonin and that carbohydrates administered during acute stress may stave off some of the worst effects. To test this hypothesis, twenty-four subjects high in stress-proneness were compared with twenty-four low in stress-proneness. The plasma ratio of tryptophan to other large neutral amino acids (LNAA) allowed for approximation for brain levels of tryptophan and serotonin. (Tryptophan is the precursor to serotonin.) As predicted, a carbohydrate-rich diet was significantly better at preventing depression and performance deterioration than the protein-rich diet for highly stress-prone subjects. This was not true for subjects low in stress-proneness.

Wurtman and colleagues (2003) also found that protein-rich versus carbohydrate-rich foods create significantly different tryptophan-to-LNAA ratios and tyrosine-to-LNAA ratios (the precursors of the neurotransmitters dopamine and norepinephrine). So carbohydrates may influence these neurotransmitters as well.

Stress can also influence choice of food and amount eaten. In a study of fifty-nine healthy premenopausal women, Epel, Lapidus, McEwen, and Brownell (2001) studied whether high cortisol reactivity was related to eating after stress. They found that women who were high cortisol reactors ate more calories after stress than low reactors. High reactors also ate significantly more sweet foods across days. Increases in negative mood as a reaction to stress also resulted in significant food consumption.

Another study of stress and eating specifically examined whether carbohydrate-rich/protein-poor foods diminished depressed mood and a cortisol response in conditions of controllable and uncontrollable stress (Markus, Panhuysen, Tuiten, & Koppeschaar, 2000). With highly stress-prone subjects, depression and cortisol levels improved, indicating that the carbohydrate-rich/protein-poor diet was increasing their ability to cope with stress. These findings suggest that carbohydrates enhanced serotonin function in highly stress-prone subjects.

What Women Can Do

Women can help control their moods by eating carbohydrates. To achieve an antidepressant effect, patients must consume at least 45 grams of either simple or complex carbohydrates with no (or very little) protein. If women want to try this approach to treating depression, Judith Wurtman's book *The Serotonin Solution* is a good resource (Wurtman & Suffes, 1997). It is written for a lay audience, and Wurtman offers specific instructions about how often to eat carbohydrates and in what amounts. This book even has a "stressed-mommy" diet, including a special "will-this-day-never-end?" diet. The focus of the book is on weight loss, but it includes a wealth of information, written in an accessible style, on the connection between food and emotions. This diet has no impact on breastfeeding.

The final point is that good nutrition, even if not done for a specific antidepressant effect, is important to mental health. It provides a feeling of physical well-being and the energy to accomplish tasks. In talking with mothers about what they eat, it may be necessary to brainstorm with them about how they can eat more nutritiously. Some suggestions include having high-nutrition snacks, such as fruits, vegetables, low-fat cheese, or yogurt, readily available. This may involve preparing snacks when someone else is available to care for the baby (such as in the evening to eat the next day). Mothers of newborns often find that they have only "one hand" during the day, so it may take some planning on the mother's part to make sure her nutritional needs are addressed.

SUPPLEMENTS

Supplements are another important treatment alternative for depression. In this chapter, I describe two types of nutritional supplements: omega-3 fatty acids and SAMe (S-adenosyl-L-methionine). A number of recent studies have found that both are effective treatments for depression (Preston & Johnson, 2004).

Omega-3 Fatty Acids

For almost 100 years, major depression in the general population has increased substantially. One theory about why this has occurred has to do with changes in our consumption of fats. Over the same time period, we have increased the amount of saturated fatty acids and decreased the amount of polyunsaturated fatty acids in our diets. Of the polyunsaturated fats, people in our culture now eat more omega-6 fatty acids (e.g., corn oil) and fewer omega-3s than we did 100 years ago, and the change in the ratio of the polyunsaturated fats is also a problem (Maes & Smith, 1998; Peet, Murphy, Shay, & Horrobin, 1998). Omega-3 fatty acids are long-chain polyunsaturated fatty acids found in plant and marine sources. They have many health benefits and are showing promise as a treatment for depression, bipolar disorder, and schizophrenia (Freeman, 2000; Stoll et al., 1999).

Why Omega-3s May Influence Depression

There are a number of theories about why omega-3s might have an influence on depression. One proposed mechanism relates to immune system function and the production of cytokines, particularly interleukin-1β (IL-1β), IL-2, and IL-6 (Maes & Smith, 1998). Cytokines are involved in depression a variety of ways. First, they provoke symptoms identical to those of major depression in humans (e.g., lethargy, social withdrawal). Second, they activate the hypothalamic-pituitary-adrenal axis, raising cortisol levels. Cortisol levels are often elevated in depression. Third, IL-1 and IL-6 lower serum concentrations of tryptophan (the precursor to serotonin) and alter brain metabolism of serotonin. Fourth, antidepressants suppress cytokines, suggesting that these medications are also anti-inflammatory. Finally, cytokines are released in response to internal and external stressors. The postpartum period is one internal stressor known to increase cytokine release. Others include infection, injury, autoimmune disease, and cancer. Omega-3s reduce cytokine production, whereas omega-6s increase it. Simopoulos (2002) noted that major depression and several physical illnesses (coronary heart disease, cancer, arthritis, Crohn's disease, ulcerative colitis, and lupus erythematosis) all feature high levels of IL-1.

Severus, Littman, and Stoll (2001) described how depression may be due to another inflammatory substance: homocysteine. Their review was concerned with the issue of why depression is related to increased rates of cardiovascular morbidity. They hypothesized that patients who suffer from both cardiovascular disease and depression often have elevated homocysteine levels and a deficiency of omega-3s.

EPA, DHA, and Depression

With regard to depression, two omega-3s are of interest: eicosapentaenoic acid (EPA) and docosahexaenoic acid (DHA). Peet et al. (1998) tested the hypothesis that depression is associated with depleted red blood cell membrane levels of total n3 fatty acids, particularly DHA. They compared the fatty acid composition in red blood cell membranes of fifteen people who were depressed (and currently medication free) and fifteen matched controls. As predicted, they found that depressed patients had significantly lower levels of polyunsaturated fatty acids, particularly DHA. Moreover, the red blood cell membranes of depressed people show oxidative damage, and this could be due to increased oxidative stress or deficient defense mechanisms.

Another study (Hibbeln et al., 1998) found that people with low serum polyunsaturated fatty acids had low levels of the metabolites of serotonin and dopamine in their cerebral spinal fluid. Lower levels of metabolites correspond to lower levels of the neurotransmitters.

Omega-3s have been used to treat depression. Ethyl-eicosapentaenoate was used in a double-blind trial to treat depression that had been resistant to treatment with standard medications (Peet & Horrobin, 2002). The authors found a significantly greater effect of EPA on depression than the placebo. At the end of the twelve-week study, patients who took EPA were significantly improved on all measures of depression, anxiety, sleep, lassitude, libido, and suicidality. One gram of EPA per day was the most effective dose. Two and four grams were only marginally effective. A case study of a severely depressed and suicidal males showed similar results (Puri, Counsell, Hamilton, Richardson, & Horrobin, 2001). This patient had been treatment resistant, with near-constant suicidal ideations. When ethyl-EPA was added to his treatment regimen, he had dramatic improvement on all symptoms within one month.

Omega-3s have also been studied in postpartum women. In one study (Hibbeln, 2002), mothers who consumed high amounts of seafood during pregnancy and had high levels of DHA in their milk had lower levels of postpartum depression than mothers who consumed low amounts of seafood and had low amounts of DHA in their milk (Hibbeln, 2002). These data were collected from 14,532 subjects, over forty-one studies. Hibbeln compared DHA, EPA, and arachidonic acid (AA) content in mothers' milk to seafood consumption rates in published reports from twenty-three countries. Hibbeln found that higher concentrations of DHA and greater seafood consumption both predicted lower prevalence rates of postpartum depression. AA and EPA were not related to rates of postpartum depression.

In another study, mothers who had higher DHA at one and two days postpartum had infants who slept better than infants of mothers low in DHA. These babies slept better because infants of high-DHA mothers had greater central nervous system maturity; DHA is essential for the baby's developing central nervous system (Cheruku, Montgomery-Downs, Farkas, Thoman, & Lammi-Keefe, 2002). Babies who are more mature sleepers also contribute to their mothers' mental health by allowing their mothers to get some much-needed sleep.

Omega-3s have also been used to treat bipolar disorder (Stoll et al., 1999). In this study, thirty patients with bipolar disorder were assigned to receive either omega-3s or a placebo in addition to their usual treatment and were followed for four months. Patients receiving the omega-3s had a significantly longer period of remission than those who received the placebo.

How to Get Omega-3s

As indicated earlier, getting omega-3s from food can ease depression. Another population study from New Zealand found that fish consumption was related to higher self-reported mental health. This study controlled for possible confounds including age, household income, eating patterns, alcohol use, and smoking. The authors felt their findings provided indirect support for the relationship between omega-3s and mood stabilization (Silvers & Scott, 2002).

There is, however, some concern about mercury contamination in seafood as it can have a significant impact on a baby's developing nervous system. Pregnant and lactating women must be careful but do not have to avoid all seafood. New Hampshire has one of the highest levels of mercury contamination in the United States. A listing of mercury-related Web sites is presented in Exhibit 9.1.

EXHIBIT 9.1. Resources for information on Mercury Contamination in Fish

U.S. Food and Drug Administration Center for Food Safety and Applied Nutrition

Food Information Line, twenty-four hours per day, 1 (888) SAFEFOOD
<http://www.cfsan.fda.gov/~dms/admehg.html>

Environmental Protection Agency

<www.epa.gov/ost/fish>

The National Listing of Fish and Wildlife Advisories (NLFWA) Database

This database includes all available information describing state, tribal, and federally issued fish consumption advisories in the United States for the fifty states, the District of Columbia, and four U.S. territories, and in Canada for the twelve provinces and territories. The database contains information provided to the EPA by the states, tribes, territories, and Canada.
<http://map1.epa.gov/>

Source: Compiled 2003 by Melissa Bernardin, Mercury Outreach Coordinator, Clean Water Fund, Portsmouth, NH. Used with permission.

Fish oil supplements are another common way to receive EPA and DHA. However, some people worry about the fishy smell or about contaminants in seafood. Again, this is a real concern for pregnant and lactating women. The amount of contaminants in a particular brand may be impossible to determine. The key is to use pharmaceutical-grade omega-3s. Exhibit 9.2 lists three manufacturers of pharmaceutical-grade fish oil supplements. These companies regularly test for contaminants including mercury and PCBs. All are available directly to consumers.

Uncontaminated fish oil appears safe and does not interact with other medications. Contrary to earlier reports, it also does not increase patient bleeding, even when combined with aspirin (Harkness & Bratman, 2003). It has no apparent impact on breastfeeding.

Vegetarians may have additional concerns about consuming an animal product. Many have turned to flaxseed as an alternative. However, the principal omega-3 in flaxseed is alpha-linolenic acid (ALA). ALA is metabolically farther removed from EPA and DHA. Supplementation with ALA does not appear to increase EPA and DHA levels and appears to have no impact on depression (Bratman & Girman, 2003). It does, however, have other beneficial effects on cardiovascular health. (The processing of flaxseed oil makes it a different supplement than flaxseed, and it is not a good source of omega-3s; see Bratman & Girman, 2003).

S-Adenosyl-L-Methionine

SAMe is another supplement that is effective in treating depression. It is a substance that naturally occurs in the body and is crucial to cell metabolism in all animals. It is derived from the amino acid methionine and adenosine triphosphate. Our bodies manufacture methionine from protein. SAMe contributes to a process known as methylation that regulates serotonin, melatonin, dopamine, and adrenaline. It also regulates neurotransmitter metabolism, membrane fluidity, and receptor activity (Bratman & Girman, 2003). If people have low levels of B_6, B_{12}, or folic acid, SAMe breaks down into homocysteine. High homocysteine levels are harmful to cardiovascular health and have been related to depression. Moreover, high levels of homocysteine during pregnancy raise the risk of spina bifida and other birth defects.

A meta-analysis of twenty-eight studies indicated that SAMe decreased depression significantly more than a placebo, and it was comparable to antidepressant medications in its effectiveness (Agency for Healthcare Research and Quality, 2002). The authors of this report noted that in placebo trials, SAMe was in fact providing an active

treatment. Clinically, patients improved, but SAMe did not completely eradicate depression.

SAMe has also been used to treat postpartum depression (Cerutti,
Sichel, & Perin, 1993). In this study, women were randomly assigned
to receive 1,600 mg of SAMe, a placebo, or usual care. By the tenth
day, women receiving SAMe had significantly lower depression scores
on the Kellner Scale than women in the placebo group. By day thirty,
however, the difference between the SAMe and placebo group was no
longer significant. The difference was still significant, however, between the women receiving SAMe and the usual-care group.

What Mothers Can Do

SAMe is generally very well tolerated. The standard dose is 200
mg twice a day, with rapid titration upward over the next one to two
weeks. It may take as much as 1,600 mg per day to achieve an initial
response in depression, but a maintenance dose can be as low as 200
mg twice a day (Bratman & Girman, 2003). This supplement has two
downsides. First, it is expensive. Even at discount stores, SAMe can
cost as much as $1.00 per pill. This cost can be prohibitive for many.
Second, SAMe degrades easily. Consumers have no way of knowing
whether the SAMe they purchased was handled correctly. Consequently, consumers may pay top dollar for an inert substance.

At this time, its impact on breastfeeding is also unknown. Since it
naturally occurs in the body it is most likely safe, but there is no research to confirm this. It is used to treat cholestasis of pregnancy
(Agency for Healthcare Research and Quality, 2002). Similarly, Bratman and Girman (2003) noted that SAMe has been used in studies of
pregnant women with no ill effects. But no one has established maximum safe doses for pregnant or lactating women.

In summary, omega-3s and SAMe both show promise for treating
postpartum depression. These supplements appear to be safe for
pregnancy and lactation, but some concerns still linger, especially
concerning contaminated seafood (and fish oil supplements).

EXERCISE

Exercise is another option that is gaining in popularity for the treatment of depression. It works because it also changes brain chemistry.

Specifically, exercise elevates serotonin and dopamine levels and releases endorphins that relieve pain and create a sense of well-being. Both aerobic and strength-training types of exercise will achieve this effect. Traditionally, exercise has been recommended for people with mild to moderate depression, but exercise can be effective for people with major depression as well. It can also be combined with other modalities to increase the effectiveness of each.

Exercise for Depressed People

Several studies have demonstrated the effectiveness of exercise in boosting mood. In a large study from Finland ($N = 3,403$), exercise lowered depression and helped with feelings of anger, distrust, and stress. Two to three times a week was enough to achieve this mood-altering effect (Hassmen, Koivula, & Uutela, 2000). Men and women who exercised perceived their health and fitness as better than non-exercisers, and this has been associated with lower levels of depression. Exercise also increased feelings of social integration.

In a study of seventy women with fibromyalgia, Da Costa, Dobkin, Dritsa, and Fitzcharles (2001) examined the relationship between depressed mood and weekly exercise. Women were evaluated at baseline and three years later. The authors found that women who engaged in more weekly leisure activity had lower depressed mood at the three-year follow-up.

Subjects randomly assigned to a twelve-week fitness program had significantly improved depression, anxiety, and self-concept at the end of the twelve weeks compared with subjects in the control group ($N = 82$, ages eighteen to thirty-nine). These findings were still true at the one year follow-up (DiLorenzo et al., 1999). In a study of sedentary, ethnic minority women, participants in the exercise group reported significant decreases in depressed mood and significant increases in vigor compared to women who did not exercise (Lee et al., 2001).

Subjects in the previously cited studies had mild to moderate depression. But Babyak et al.'s (2000) study demonstrated that exercise can be helpful for major depression too. The subjects in this study were randomly assigned to three groups: exercise alone, sertraline (Zoloft) alone, or a combinanation of exercise and sertraline. All subjects improved after four months. There were also no differences between the groups, indicating that people in the exercise-only group did as well as people in the two medication groups. Combining medications with exercise did not improve the intervention. The rates of relapse are also of interest. Six months after completion of treatment, the exercise group had lower rates of relapse. Subjects who continued to exercise after the end of treatment had lower risk of depression. The authors concluded that exercise is helpful, even in subjects with major depression.

Researchers usually explain the lower relapse rates in exercise (or cognitive therapy) groups by noting that these modalities give people tools to cope with life's stresses. Conversely, when people are on medication alone, and the medication is gone, they are no better off in terms of coping than before they started their treatment. On the other hand, medication may be necessary to help patients get the maximum benefit from other interventions.

In a sample of thirty-two elders (ages sixty to eighty-four years), subjects were randomized to one of two conditions; ten weeks of supervised weight-lifting exercise followed by ten weeks of unsupervised exercise. The control subjects attended lectures for ten weeks. The subjects all had major or minor depression. The researchers had no contact with any study participant until the end of the research period at twenty-six months. Subjects in the exercise group had significantly lower scores on the Beck Depression Inventory at twenty weeks, and at follow-up at twenty-six months, than the nonexercisers. Moreover, at the twenty-six-month follow-up, 33 percent of the exercisers were still regularly lifting weights versus 0 percent of the controls (Singh, Clements, & Fiatarone Singh, 2001).

In another sample of older adults, patients were randomly assigned to either exercise classes or health education for ten weeks (Mather et al., 2002). All subjects were depressed, but their depression was not adequately controlled by medication. Exercise was proposed as an adjunct to treatment. Blind assessments were made before the study started, and at ten and thirty-four weeks. In the sample, 55 percent of the exercise group improved their depression score on the Hamilton Rating Scale for Depression by 30 percent, compared with only 33 percent of the group who received education.

The mood-altering effects of exercise appear fairly quickly. In a study of twenty-six women, Lane, Crone-Grant, and Lane (2002) measured anger, confusion, depression, fatigue, tension, and vigor before and after two exercise sessions. Significant mood enhancement occurred after each exercise session. Depressed mood was especially sensitive to exercise, and decreased significantly after each session.

Exercise and Breastfeeding

One concern mothers may raise is the impact of exercise on breastfeeding. Does exercise cause lactic acid to build in their milk so babies will not take it? Or, worse, is it actually harmful for babies? A study of twelve lactating women sought to answer this question (Quinn & Carey, 1999). In this study, milk and blood samples were taken after a nonexercise session (control), after maximal exercise, and after a session that was 20 percent below the maximal range. They found that in women with an adequate maternal caloric intake, moderate exercise did not increase lactic acid in breast milk. Increases occurred when women were exercising in a range that they considered "hard" (using the perceived-exertion scale). The authors recommended, therefore, exercise in a moderate range. So moderate exercise does not appear to alter babies' willingness to breastfeed, nor is it harmful to babies.

What Mothers Can Do

Exercise can be helpful treatment for depression and can be used in combination with other treatment modalities. To achieve an antidepressant effect, mothers should exercise at least two to three times a week for at least twenty minutes. In working with mothers, it is important to let them know about exercise's impact on brain chemistry. Otherwise, it will be the last thing that they feel like doing. For most mothers, it will be helpful if they can work it naturally into their day rather than trying to set aside a block of time (which somehow never materializes). In summary, exercise can be highly effective and offers mothers an alternative to medications.

COMBINED MODALITIES AND OTHER TECHNIQUES

At this point, a large empirical base on the efficacy of other alternative treatments for postpartum depression is lacking. However, a review highlights that some of the approaches are promising and should be considered as possible treatments for depressed mothers. Some of these other modalities include Ayurvedic medicine, homeopathy, aromatherapy, massage, and traditional Chinese medicine (Mantle, 2002). According to the House of Lords' Select Committee on Science and Technology (2000) report, all of these have at least some evidence base for treating depression, with the exceptions of traditional Chinese and Ayurvedic medicine.

Combining multiple modalities also has a synergistic effect. In a study of 112 women (ages nineteen to seventy-eight) with mild to moderate depression, walking outside in the sun twenty minutes a day plus taking a vitamin supplement decreased depression and improved overall mood, self-esteem, and general sense of well-being (Brown, Goldstein-Shirley, Robinson, & Casey, 2001). The inclusion of sunlight in this study design is interesting. Especially for those of us in northern climates, lack of sunlight can be a big factor in depression, particularly for women who have babies during the winter. Except for one published case study (described next), the effects of sunlight have not been studied with postpartum women. But some mothers report that it is helpful to get outside for at least a little time each day.

Bright light was helpful in an article describing two case studies of new mothers (Corral, Kuan, & Kostaras, 2000). In this article, two new mothers became suddenly depressed after the birth of their babies. They refused to take antidepressants but agreed to a trial of bright light therapy. Both of these women responded to bright light therapy and had significantly lower rates of depressive symptoms after treatment.

In a Finnish study of healthy adults (ages twenty-six to sixty-three years), patients were randomly assigned to three conditions: aerobics class with bright light, aerobics class with normal illumination, and relaxation/stretching sessions in bright light as a control group. The study period lasted for eight weeks. The authors found that bright light and exercise relieved depression. For atypical depression, bright light was more effective than exercise. The authors concluded that twice-weekly administration of bright light, alone or with physical exercise, could alleviate seasonal depression (Leppaemaeki, Partonen, Hurme, Haukka, & Loennqvist, 2002).

In a review, Manber, Allen, and Morris (2002) noted that exercise, stress reduction, bright light exposure, and sleep deprivation might be more effective as adjuncts to traditional treatment than as treatments by themselves. They also noted preliminary evidence suggesting that acupuncture might be helpful in the treatment of single-episode major depression.

CONCLUSION

Diet, supplements, and exercise are all effective treatments for depression—even major depression. These modalities are also low-cost (except for SAMe), not harmful, and mothers can initiate them themselves. They also have the advantage of having a minimal impact on breastfeeding. They can be combined with traditional treatment, or offered as an alternative to mothers who refuse to take medications. As with other treatments for depression, mothers should be monitored to determine whether these techniques are reducing their depression. If not, other options should be added or used instead.

In the next chapter, I describe community-based interventions and two types of psychotherapy that have proven effective for the treatment of depression in new mothers.

·Chapter 10

Community Interventions
and Psychotherapy

In this chapter, I describe psychotherapy and interventions that involve community support and education for mothers. The knowledge base on community support and interpersonal psychotherapy is still new enough that some gaps exist. Cognitive-behavioral therapy (CBT), in contrast, has a large body of empirical support and has been shown to be as effective as medications. I have also included a discussion of trauma-focused therapy for mothers who have suffered past or current trauma. I write these sections aware that you may not be providing this therapy yourself. But you may be making referrals to others who do. Understanding the full range of options available will help you direct mothers to the services they need.

COMMUNITY INTERVENTIONS

In an article on integrative care for women suffering from postpartum depression, LoCicero, Weiss, and Issokson (1997) state that effective treatment and prevention efforts involve understanding women in their context of their social and community networks. They proposed that communities coordinate a network of services and resources and make these available to childbearing families. The authors recommended routine screening for postpartum depression, interdisciplinary coordination and referral, and improvement in provision of perinatal health care.

Efficacy of Community-Based Care

Community-based care has been effective for postpartum women. In a study of 2,064 women, half were assigned to an intervention of flexible care provided by midwives, and the other half were assigned to standard care. At four months postpartum, women in the flexible-care group had significantly better mental health than women in the standard-care group. The authors concluded that midwife-led, flexible care that was tailored to individual needs significantly improved new mothers' mental health and reduced the risk of postpartum depression (MacArthur et al., 2002).

In a Scottish study, women in midwife-managed care had lower scores on the EPDS seven weeks after birth than women who received standard care (Shields, Reid, & Cheyne, 1997). Similarly, in Australia, women identified as at risk for child abuse and neglect received structured home visits soon after birth or were in the control group. At six weeks postpartum, women in the intervention group had significantly lower rates of postpartum depression (Armstrong et al., 1999).

A study from England had different results. This study sought to determine whether additional support in the first month postpartum increased maternal health and breastfeeding rates and decreased the risk of postpartum depression (Morrell, Spiby, Stewart, Walters, & Morgan, 2000). There were 623 women in the study. Half were assigned to receive home visits, and the other half were assigned to receive standard care. At six weeks postpartum, there were no significant differences in health status, use of social services, or depression or breastfeeding rates. The mothers were very satisfied with the health visits, however.

A study from South Africa found improvement in mother-infant interaction, but not in depression, after a home visiting program (Cooper et al., 2002). In this study, thirty-two women were randomly assigned to receive home visits by trained community volunteers, and they were compared with a matched group of thirty-two women who received usual care. The home visitors provided emotional support and taught mothers to be more responsive to their babies using items from the Neonatal Behavioral Assessment Scale. This intervention had no significant impact on maternal mood (although it was better for mothers in the intervention group) but was significantly associated with mothers being more positive with their babies.

Community-based care even helps in the general population. Simon, VonKorff, Rutter, and Wagner (2000) found that telephone follow-up by a care manager significantly improved patient compliance with antidepressant treatment. This resulted in a 50 percent improvement in depression scores and a lower probability of major depression at the six-month follow-up than standard care. The telephone follow-up consisted of a five-minute introductory telephone call and two ten- to fifteen-minute calls at eight and sixteen weeks after the initial prescription. The case managers also communicated with doctors about whether there were side effects, or whether the patient might be undermedicated (i.e., still showing moderate levels of depression). The case managers also assisted with arrangements for follow-up visits, but did not provide psychotherapy.

Education

Education is a key component of many community-based programs that aim to reduce the risk of depression and help mothers have more positive interactions with their babies. The results on the effectiveness of these programs, however, have been mixed. In one education program (Elliot et al., 2000), women identified during pregnancy as being vulnerable to depression were randomly assigned to a preventive intervention or a control group. At three months postpartum, 19 percent of the women in the Preparation for Parenthood group had scores in the depressed or borderline depressed ranges compared with 39 percent of the mothers who received standard care. These findings were true only for first-time mothers.

Another study found that education during pregnancy was not helpful in reducing postpartum depression (Hayes, Muller, & Bradley, 2001). In this study, women were randomly assigned to either an education condition or normal care. Depression was assessed during pregnancy and at two points postpartum. There were no differences between the control and intervention groups. Furthermore, social support or demographic variables had no relevant influence. Depressive symptoms for both groups improved over time: both were more likely to be depressed during pregnancy than at either point postpartum. The authors concluded that their findings challenge two beliefs strongly held by professionals in the perinatal health field: first, that depression can be reduced through education; and second, that interventions during pregnancy can endure into the postpartum period.

In summary, community-based programs show promise in helping women make a smooth transition to motherhood. However, these programs must take place alongside more traditional, individually focused interventions for depression. Moreover, we need research that demonstrates the effectiveness of these programs in preventing or ameliorating postpartum depression.

PSYCHOTHERAPY

Psychotherapy encompasses two types of treatment for depression: CBT and interpersonal psychotherapy (IPT). Both types have shown effectiveness in treating depressed mothers.

Cognitive-Behavioral Therapy

One highly effective type of psychotherapy for depression is CBT. CBT has proven to be as powerful as medications for treating depression, anxiety, chronic pain, and OCD (Antonuccio, 1995). Moreover, patients who received CBT did better on follow-up, were less likely to relapse, and were less likely to drop out of treatment than those who received medications alone (Antonuccio, 1995; Antonuccio, Danton, & DeNelsky, 1995).

CBT is based on the premise that depression is caused by distortions in thinking. The goal is to help patients learn to identify distorted beliefs and replace them with more rational ones. CBT is not simply learning to think happy thoughts.

A review (DeRubeis, Gelfand, Tang, & Simons, 1999) had similar findings. DeRubeis and colleagues compared the results of four randomized trials on the efficacy of medication versus CBT for severely depressed patients. The effect sizes comparing antidepressants to CBT favored the therapy. But when tests compared medications versus CBT, there was no significant difference between the two.

Cognitive therapy can also change the brain. The impact of cognitive therapy on the brain can be seen in a study of OCD (Baxter, Schwartz, Bergman, & Szuba, 1992). Patients with OCD were randomly assigned to receive either medication or cognitive therapy. Before therapy, both groups had positron emission tomography (PET) scans, and patients in both groups showed abnormalities in brain metabolism. After treatment, both groups had better PET scans than they did before treatment. However, there was no difference between the groups. In other words, cognitive therapy caused the same changes in the brain that medications had.

CBT has also been used to assist new mothers with postpartum depression. In a study from England, eighty-seven postpartum women with depressive illness were randomly assigned to one of four conditions: fluoxetine (Prozac) or placebo, plus one or six sessions of CBT (Appleby, Warner, Whitton, & Faragher, 1997). Health visitors who attended a brief training provided the CBT. The sessions were designed to offer reassurance and advice on areas of concern to new mothers. The initial session was one hour, and subsequent sessions were thirty minutes each. Four weeks after treatment, all four groups had improved. Not surprisingly, women receiving fluoxetine improved significantly more than women receiving the placebo, and women receiving six sessions of counseling improved significantly more than women who only received one session. There was no advantage for women receiving both medication and counseling beyond the first session. CBT was as effective as medication.

We should not be too optimistic about what general practitioners can do in terms of cognitive therapy, however. In a clinical trial, general practitioners and patients with depression or anxiety were randomly assigned to intervention or control groups. Physicians in the intervention group attended sixteen hours of sessions on brief cognitive therapy (King et al., 2002). Six months later, there was no difference between trained and nontrained physicians in their knowledge and attitudes about depression. There were no effects on patient outcomes as well.

Problem Solving

A subtype of cognitive therapy is problem solving. This approach was effective in two randomized trials of primary-care patients with major depression (Mynors-Wallis, Gath, Day & Baker, 2000; Mynors-Wallis, Gath, Lloyd-Thomas, & Tomlinson, 1995). The first study included ninety-one primary care patients with major depression. They were assigned to the problem-solving treatment, amitriptyline plus standard clinical management, or a placebo with standard clinical management. After twelve weeks, patients in the problem-solving and medication groups were significantly less depressed than patients in the placebo group. There was no significant difference in depression between those in the medication versus problem-solving groups. These sessions were administered by a general practitioner and focused on how patients could effectively solve a particular problem that they identified in the first session. Patients were encouraged to define and clarify their problems, generate solutions, choose achievable goals, and evaluate whether their efforts paid off (Mynors-Wallis et al., 1995).

A general practice nurse provided the problem-solving intervention in the second study (Mynors-Wallis et al., 2000). The medications in this study were fluvoxamine or paroxetine. Patients were assigned to medication alone or a combination of problem solving with medication. The authors found that nurses could deliver this intervention as well as physicians. Again, problem solving alone was as effective as medication. There was no increased effect of combining medication with problem solving.

What Mothers Can Do

Mothers who are interested in cognitive therapy have at least two options. The first is to read the book *Feeling Good: The New Mood Therapy* by psychiatrist David Burns. Burns (1999) addresses ten types of cognitive distortions that are common and lists specific strategies for dealing with them. It is do-it-yourself cognitive therapy. This book can be a great resource for patients, especially those who are motivated to try this approach and like to read. If mothers are looking for a practitioner, they can contact their local state psychological association or go to Burns' Web site (www.feelinggood.com) for a listing of providers.

As a note of caution, it is advisable to proceed gently when working with mothers. Once you become aware of cognitive distortions, you will see them everywhere. Many times, we can help a mother reframe the situation more positively, focusing on what she can do. But if she is in real distress, we must be careful not to dismiss her concerns just because we hear a cognitive distortion behind them.

Interpersonal Psychotherapy

IPT is another type of psychotherapy that has proven effective in the treatment of depression. In a National Institutes of Mental Health collaborative research study, IPT was as effective as tricyclic anti-depressants and cognitive therapy and was effective for almost 70 percent of the patients (Tolman, 2001).

IPT is based on attachment theory and the interpersonal theories of Harry Stack Sullivan. It is time limited, and focuses on the client's interpersonal relationships. Disturbances in these relationships are hypothesized as being responsible for depression in general and postpartum depression in particular (Stuart & O'Hara, 1995). In IPT, there are four problem areas: role transitions, interpersonal disputes, grief, and interpersonal deficits. On a client's first visit, a specific problem is identified, and the client and therapist begin work on that issue. Stuart and O'Hara noted that in their experience, postpartum depression is related to role transitions. The goal of IPT is to help new mothers combine their new roles with the ones they have already established. This might involve helping the mother solve a problem. But the actual solution is less important than the process of identifying a problem and making a change.

In a pilot study, Stuart and O'Hara (1995) found that six depressed women who completed twelve weeks of IPT were all significantly less depressed than when they began: none met criteria for major depression by the study's end. There was no comparison group in this preliminary study.

In a larger study of 120 women with postpartum major depression (O'Hara, Stuart, Gorman, & Wenzel, 2000), women were assigned to either interpersonal psychotherapy or wait-list conditions for twelve weeks. The therapists were highly trained in IPT, and they followed a standardized treatment manual. O'Hara et al. found that women in the therapy group had significantly lower depression scores than women in the wait-list group at four, eight, and twelve weeks after the completion of treatment. The rate of recovery from depression was also significantly higher for women in the therapy group, and they scored better on postpartum adjustment and social support. The authors noted that interpersonal therapy was effective for women with postpartum depression. IPT reduced depressive symptoms and improved social adjustment. The authors felt that IPT represents a viable alternative to pharmacotherapy, especially for women who are breastfeeding.

Klier, Muzik, Rosenblum, and Lenz (2001) also found IPT effective for seventeen women with postpartum depression. In this case, the IPT was used in group therapy. Women had significantly decreased depression after attending the group, and this was still true at the six-month follow-up. The authors noted some limitations in their study, such as small sample size, lack of a control group, and possible bias in the therapist's assessment of the women.

In summary, CBT and IPT are both effective treatments for postpartum depression. At this time, there is more empirical support for CBT. Mothers may have an easier time locating a practitioner who can provide CBT. But IPT shows a lot of promise and hopefully will be the focus of future studies.

TRAUMA-FOCUSED TREATMENT

The final type of treatment I describe is trauma-focused treatment. Women may come into the postpartum period with significant trauma, which may be related to current events such as their childbirth experiences, events that took place in the past, or both. Trauma treatment involves a combination of patient education, peer counseling, medications, and psychotherapy. (Medications for PTSD are described in the next chapter.) The combination of all these modalities provides the best overall care. Patient education, peer counseling, and psychotherapy are described in this section.

Since the recognition of trauma in postpartum women is relatively new, no studies specifically address postpartum PTSD. However, many studies from the general trauma literature have addressed the efficacy of these techniques. These studies are summarized next.

Patient Education

Women who have been traumatized by childbirth events, past abuse, or other events are often frightened by their reactions. Education is the first component of a treatment plan. It can reassure women that they are not going crazy, which many actually fear, and lets them know that they are not alone in their reactions. Patient education contains four key elements: normalization, removing self-blame and doubt, correcting misunderstandings, and establishing clinician credibility (Friedman, 2001).

Normalization

Normalization lets women know that their symptoms are similar to those experienced by millions of people who have been through traumatic events. This can create a profound sense of relief. Women learn that there is no stigma attached to their reactions, nor are they a result of weakness. Rather, normalization communicates that PTSD is a common human response to trauma.

Removing Self-Blame and Self-Doubt

Many survivors of traumatic events blame themselves for being in harm's way and are ashamed that they did not take some kind of heroic steps to avoid the trauma or get out of the dangerous circumstance. This can be behind the second guessing that mothers will do following childbirth or other traumatic events. They may lament that they "should have known better." Education can help patients realize that they did the best they could under the circumstances and with the information that was available. Patient education can also help women evaluate how realistic their heroic fantasies are. It can communicate that their "failure" to act was due to the overwhelming nature of the event itself.

Correcting Misunderstandings

Patient education, and education of family members and friends, can help people understand a woman's behaviors in terms of PTSD. Behaviors that seem strange or upsetting can be explained in light of the woman's experiences. This can help those in her support network work with, rather than against, treatment goals. It can also help women recover from previous traumatic events.

Clinician Credibility

Finally, patient education can help establish you as knowledgeable about trauma, and can show that you understand what women are experiencing. This helps in enlisting women's cooperation in treatment and can facilitate the development of trust.

The Efficacy of Patient Education

At this point, there has been no study of patient education alone in the treatment of PTSD. This is because education is never used alone. It is always an adjunct to other treatment modalities (Friedman, 2001). However, most clinicians agree that it is an important component of any type of therapeutic approach.

Peer Counseling

Peer counseling uses an approach similar to that of Alcoholics Anonymous, in that everyone involved in the group has had personal experience with trauma and PTSD and wants to take more control over his or her life. Some examples of postpartum peer counseling groups could include groups for women who had cesarean or other difficult childbirths, mothers of premature or ill infants, mothers who have experienced previous childbearing loss, and mothers who are abuse survivors. The relationships in the peer group are equalitarian, and no authority figure or professional leads the group. Sometimes a therapist who is treating several women with similar experiences may bring them together for a few sessions. These groups can also take place on the Internet. Peer counselors often serve as role models for new clients and demonstrate that it is possible to move beyond traumatic experiences (Friedman, 2001).

The Efficacy of Peer Counseling

Peer counseling has not been studied for its effectiveness since the very nature of the peer group tends to limit professional involvement. However, anecdotal and clinical reports indicate that these groups can have a positive effect on participants and can be a useful component of treatment (Friedman, 2001).

Trauma-Focused Psychotherapy

When women have been traumatized, their bodies and minds develop a conditioned response that pairs the traumatic event with certain environmental cues (e.g., sights, sounds, smells) and bodily sensations (e.g., pain). This is known as fear conditioning. In trauma-focused psychotherapy, the first goal is to unlearn the conditioned response that triggers PTSD symptoms. The second is to address PTSD-related cognitions.

Psychotherapy is generally the treatment of choice for people with PTSD. Two of the most effective individual treatments are CBT, and eye movement desensitization and reprocessing (EMDR). These techniques are described next.

Cognitive-Behavioral Therapy

CBT is designed to counteract conditioned fear responses and to normalize abnormal thoughts, behaviors, and feelings of patients with PTSD. Of the several types of CBT, some are more effective than others. Three popular forms of CBT are exposure therapy, cognitive therapy, and stress-inoculation training.

Exposure therapy. Exposure therapy is specifically designed to alleviate the conditioned emotional response to traumatic stimuli. After a traumatic event, patients naturally tend to avoid any memories of it or any stimuli that remind them of their trauma. This behavior could cause mothers to miss follow-up appointments or refuse any contact with care providers. However, when patients avoid processing their trauma, this avoidance inhibits their recovery. Exposure therapy forces trauma survivors to confront these memories, thereby making the memories lessen their hold on patients (Foa & Cahill, 2002).

Exposure therapy begins when patients are asked to imagine the traumatic event. Patients who have experienced multiple or continuous traumatic events (such as childhood abuse) are asked to imagine the worst event that they can remember completely. Patients are asked to describe what happened, and their thoughts and feelings that occurred during the trauma, repeatedly in a single session (Foa & Cahill, 2002). During their narratives, patients are asked to report their level of distress every ten minutes. Initially, most patients are highly distressed. However, as they repeat their stories, their levels of distress tend to decrease. If treatment has been successful, then patients can confront their traumatic pasts without triggering PTSD symptoms, especially intrusive thoughts or hyperarousal. It also helps patients not generalize their anxiety to other situations that are actually safe but appear similar to the dangerous situation they were in.

Exposure therapy helps patients master their fears and counters the belief that they are weak or incompetent (Foa & Cahill, 2002). This form of treatment is highly effective and has had higher rates of success than supportive counseling (Foa & Cahill, 2002; Friedman, 2001). However, van der Kolk (2002) cautions that too much exposure to traumatic memories can backfire and actually precipitate PTSD symptoms such as hyperarousal and sensitization.

Cognitive therapy. As described earlier, cognitive therapy addresses distortions in thinking. Women who have been traumatized often see the world as a dangerous place and see themselves as helpless (Foa & Cahill, 2002; Friedman, 2001). The goal of cognitive therapy is to help patients identify these automatic thoughts and replace them with more accurate ones (Foa & Cahill, 2002). This form of therapy is also highly effective in reducing symptoms of PTSD (Friedman, 2001).

Stress-inoculation training. Stress-inoculation training (SIT) uses a combination of methods to help survivors cope with anxiety, trauma-related stimuli, and threatening situations. SIT is based on social-learning theory, which states that traumatic events create behavioral, social, and cognitive fear responses. In SIT, women learn relaxation techniques, biofeedback, cognitive restructuring, and assertiveness training to help them deal more effectively with social relationships (Friedman, 2001).

Although relaxation techniques alone have not been very effective in dealing with PTSD symptoms, they are helpful when combined with these other techniques. SIT is as effective as exposure therapy for reducing PTSD symptoms, and these improvements last over time (Friedman, 2001).

Eye Movement Desensitization and Reprocessing

EMDR is another treatment that has proven effective for many people who have experienced traumatic events. It is based on the premise that saccadic eye movements can reprogram the brain and therefore can be used to help alleviate the emotional impact of trauma. (Saccadic eye movements are quick movements as the eye jumps from one fixation point to another.)

During EMDR, women imagine a traumatic memory or any negative emotions associated with that memory. Then women are asked to articulate a belief that is incompatible with their previous memory (e.g., on their personal worth). While women are remembering this event, they are asked use their eyes to follow the clinician's fingers, which are making rapid movements. During treatment, women are asked to rate the strength of both the traumatic memory and the counteracting positive beliefs (Friedman, 2001).

Studies have demonstrated that this method of treatment is effective and has results superior to those of psychodynamic or supportive therapies. In examining the results of a number of different studies, 50 to 70 percent of patients no longer met criteria for PTSD after receiving EMDR treatment. In contrast, only 20 to 50 percent of women who received supportive therapy no longer met PTSD criteria (Friedman, 2001). However, studies on the efficacy of EMDR have some methodological limitations, including nonblind evaluations, lack of pretreatment diagnosis via a valid measure, and small sample sizes. Nevertheless, initial data suggest that this is a promising approach for the treatment of chronic PTSD (Foa & Cahill, 2002).

Interestingly, the exact mechanism for these changes remains unclear. The eye movements do not appear to have any impact on results when treatment is offered with or without eye movements (Friedman, 2001; van der Kolk, 2002). Some have hypothesized that this treatment works because of its impact on underlying cognitions, making it a form of CBT. Proponents of EMDR strongly disagree (Friedman, 2001).

The Efficacy of Psychotherapy

Overall, it appears that CBT is the most effective treatment for PTSD. Of the forms of CBT, exposure therapy has the best empirical support (Foa & Cahill, 2002). In one study that directly compared CBT to EMDR, patients assigned to the CBT group had significantly fewer symptoms posttreatment than patients assigned to EMDR. Those who received CBT were almost three times as likely to have recovered from PTSD at the three-month follow-up (Devilly & Spence, 1999). However, EMDR is also effective in treating all three clusters of symptoms and can be a useful addition to treatment regimens (Friedman, 2001). SIT has also proven effective for the treatment of rape-related PTSD. Combining psychotherapy treatments does not increase their effectiveness and may actually lessen the effectiveness of the individual treatment (Foa & Cahill, 2002). Exposure therapy appears to be most effective for those with low levels of functioning before beginning treatment, whereas SIT is helpful for patients with high levels of anxiety (Foa & Cahill, 2002). However, van der Kolk (2002) cautions that, particularly in the case of complex PTSD, many questions about optimal treatment remain. He states that what appears to be most important is to give patients a sense of mastery that will allow them to live in the present rather than the past, and to no longer be held captive by their memories.

Preventing Subsequent Childbirth-Related Trauma

When women have had traumatic experiences, they may face childbirth with fear and anxiety. This can be true for both trauma caused by childbirth events and trauma from other sources. Reynolds (1997) offers some specific suggestions for helping women with a trauma history prepare to give birth. First, good communication between the woman and her provider is essential. This will allow women to have as much control as possible, thereby reducing their anxiety. Second, since pain is often an issue and an important predictor of trauma, pain control is important. That being said, pain control must be offered while respecting women's wishes to avoid or limit medication. When dealing with trauma from a previous childbirth, Reynolds also recommended that women be asked if they felt that they or their babies were in mortal danger at any time during labor. In my experience, this is quite common, even if not medically true. As I mentioned earlier, in terms of PTSD reactions, what a mother believes is more relevant to her reaction than what is medically true. With preparation and good support, even women with substantial trauma histories can have positive, nontraumatizing childbirth experiences.

CONCLUSION

Research on treatment for postpartum depression is a new and welcome addition to the literature. But much remains to do. In a review, Lumely and Austin (2001) noted that prevention programs and interventions need strong scientific evaluation. One aspect of evaluation research is determining whether the program is being delivered as planned. Women need to exhibit a clinically relevant decrease in symptoms, and studies need to have larger sample sizes and a program that accounts for and minimizes attrition. What we have is a start, and it confirms that postpartum depression can be successfully treated with psychotherapy. In the next chapter, I summarize the final treatment option: use of antidepressant medications.

Chapter 11

Psychoactive Substances: Herbs and Antidepressants

In this chapter, I describe the efficacy of two types of antidepressants: herbal and conventional. Both are effective and have an extensive history of use in treating depression. Unlike the treatment techniques described in the previous two chapters, antidepressants have the potential to impact breastfeeding. This can be a key issue for mothers.

Much of the work I do as a lactation consultant concerns medication use and breastfeeding. My role, in that capacity, is to help mothers weigh their options and decide which approach is best for them. A few mothers may choose to wean before they take medications. They may see the choice as between "contaminated" breast milk versus "pristine" formula. But as Hale (2004) describes, this belief is not consistent with the research literature. There are known and scientifically well-established hazards associated with not breastfeeding. These hazards often outweigh risks associated with exposing infants to medication. Risks are also associated with untreated depression. Fortunately, antidepressant medication choices compatible with breastfeeding are available, so mothers usually are not forced to make this tough choice. The full range of medication options is described in this chapter.

HERBAL ANTIDEPRESSANTS

Herbal medications have a long history of use around the world and are the most common form of healing in many cultures. Despite their increasing popularity in the United States, many health care providers are uncomfortable with patients medicating themselves for something as serious as depression. To make matters worse, patients often do not tell their doctors that they are taking herbs for fear of censure. This can be dangerous because of the potential for drug interactions.

Why Patients Take Herbs

So why do patients take herbs? From the patient's perspective, herbs offer a number of advantages. If you understand why women might prefer to take herbs, it can help you talk with women about them.

- *Control:* One reason patients take herbal medications is that they can get them without a prescription and can therefore control their own health care. Instead of having to wait for a doctor's appointment, they can take care of their problem today.
- *Privacy:* Patients may be ashamed to admit that they are depressed and frightened by the possibility that their employers or others will find out that they are on antidepressants. Unfortunately, sometimes medication information is released to employers via insurance forms, and it can influence hiring and promotion decisions.
- *Costs:* Newer and name-brand antidepressants can be very expensive, especially if not covered by insurance. In contrast, herbs are generally reasonably priced and can be purchased at discount and warehouse stores. The savings each month can be substantial compared with name-brand prescription drugs.
- *Side effects:* The side effect profile is generally better with herbal medications than with standard antidepressants. The tricyclics have a host of anticholinergic side effects, including dry mouth, constipation, and blurred vision. The selective serotonin reuptake inhibitors (SSRIs) have sexual side effects such as inorgasmia. Many patients find these side effects intolerable and often stop taking their medications.

Finding Quality Herbs

Consumers are often concerned about how to know if a particular brand of herb is of good quality. Fortunately, there are some resources for finding this information. The seal of the U.S. Pharmacopeia

(USP) is one indicator of quality (see Exhibit 11.1). Companies can voluntarily submit to the criteria of the USP, and the presence of this seal ensures that these standards have been met. Exhibit 11.1 lists other information that should be on the label. Exhibit 11.2 gives the names of Web sites that rate the quality of various brands of herbs. The two most common herbs used for depression are St. John's wort and kava. These are described next.

St. John's Wort

Of the herbs used to treat depression, the one with the longest track record is St. John's wort *(Hypericum perforatum)*. It is the most widely used of the herbal antidepressants but has many other properties. It is antibacterial, anti-inflammatory, antiviral, and relieves pain (Balch, 2002; Ernst, 2002).

Use of St. John's wort dates back to the Middle Ages when it was used to treat insanity resulting from "attacks of the devil." It was named "St. John's" in reference to St. John's Day on the medieval church calendar, because it blooms near this day (June 24). *Wort* is

---

EXHIBIT 11.1.
What You Should Look for on an Herbal Product Label

Standards for Herbal Preparations

Statement of percentage of standardization of the extract
Statement describing which compounds are standardized
Statement describing which parts of the plant are used in the formulation
Extract ratio (the ratio of extract concentration to crude plant materials, e.g., 1:4)
Recommended daily dosage
Weight and number of capsules or tablets per package
Substantiated structure/function claims
Product expiration date to confirm freshness
A toll-free number and/or Web site address for company information and contact
USP: Notation that the manufacturer followed standards of the U.S. Pharmacopeia

Source: Institute for Natural Products Research. (2000). *Pocket reference guide to botanical and dietary supplements.* Marine on St. Croix, MN: Institute for Natural Products Research. Used with permission.

EXHIBIT 11.2.
Where to Go for Information on Herbs and Herb Safety

Web Sites on Herbs and Supplements

<www.ConsumerLab.com>: Rates quality of nutritional products through independent testing

<www.discoverherbs.com>: *Herbs for Health* magazine

<www.herbalgram.org>: *The Complete German Commission E Monographs,* available online and for purchase from the American Botanical Council

<www.herbal-ahp.org>: American Herbal Pharmacopoeia

<www.nccam.nih.gov>: National Center for Complementary and Alternative Medicine

---

the old English word for any medicinal plant. It is native to England, Wales, and northern Europe. Settlers brought it to North America in the 1700s (Balch, 2002), and the species now is a common wildflower in the northeastern and north central United States.

Efficacy of St. John's Wort

One burning question is whether St. John's wort actually works. The short answer is yes. Most of the earlier research was done in Germany, whose health care system uses St. John's wort extensively for the treatment of mild to moderate depression. In a meta-analysis published in the *British Medical Journal,* Linde and colleagues (1996) noted that they did not restrict their search of research studies to those published in English-language journals because there was only one. Rather, they combined the results of twenty-three randomized trials, most conducted in German-speaking countries. In this analysis, they found that hypericum extracts were significantly superior to placebos and were as effective as standard antidepressants. They indicated that the rate of study dropouts and side effects was lower for St. John's wort than antidepressants. Placebo groups (across thirteen studies) had an average response rate of 22.3 percent, compared with 55 percent of the hypericum groups.

A more recent review of twenty-two studies had similar findings (Whiskey, Werneke, & Taylor, 2001). The authors found that St. John's wort was more effective than placebo but was not significantly different from antidepressants. They also concluded that side effects were more common with standard antidepressants than with St. John's wort.

Another trial compared St. John's wort (*Hypericum perforatum* extract STEI 300) to a placebo and a tricyclic antidepressant (imipramine). The subjects were 263 primary care patients with moderate depression. The authors found that St. John's wort was effective for moderately depressed patients after four, six, and eight weeks of treatment (Philipp, Kohnen, & Hiller, 1999). They also found that St. John's wort was as effective as imipramine and that patients tolerated St. John's wort better, thereby increasing patient compliance.

In another study (Lecrubier, Clerc, Didi, & Kieser, 2002), 375 patients were randomized to receive either St. John's wort (*Hypericum perforatum* extract WS 5570) or a placebo for mild to moderate depression. The patients received treatment for six weeks. At the end of six weeks, patients receiving St. John's wort had significantly lower scores on the Hamilton Depression Rating Scale, and significantly more patients were in remission or had a response to treatment, than patients receiving the placebo. Interestingly, both groups had similar rates of adverse effects. Also, 53 percent of the patients in the St. John's wort group responded to treatment compared with 42 percent of the placebo group. The authors concluded that St. John's wort was safe and effective for the treatment of mild to moderate depression.

Unfortunately, another well-publicized study resulted in much media misinformation concerning the efficacy of St. John's wort (Hypericum Depression Trial Study Group, 2002). In this study, 340 adults with major depression were randomly assigned to receive *H. perforatum,* a placebo, or sertraline (Zoloft) for eight weeks. Subjects responding to the medication could opt to receive still-blinded treatment for another eighteen weeks. Depression was assessed at baseline and again at eight weeks. The researchers found no significant difference in depression levels or rate of response between the placebo and St. John's wort. That much was widely reported. What the media did not report was that the same was true for sertraline. The rate of full response was almost identical for the St. John's wort and sertraline groups (24 percent versus 25 percent). Eight weeks may not have been sufficient for patients with moderate to severe major depression. Neither St. John's wort nor the prescription antidepressant was effective with this group. The authors noted that their findings were not unusual in that approximately 35 percent of studies of standard antidepressants show no greater efficacy than the placebo.

Another study of patients with major depression had contrasting results. This study (van Gurp, Meterissian, Haiek, McCusker, & Bellavance, 2002) included eighty-seven patients with major depression recruited from Canadian family practice physicians. Patients were randomly assigned to receive either St. John's wort or sertraline. At the end of the twelve-week trial, both groups improved, and there was no difference between the two groups. But the sertraline group showed significantly more side effects at two and four weeks. The authors concluded that St. John's wort, because of its effectiveness and benign side effects, was a good first choice for this primary-care population.

Mechanism for Efficacy

The exact mechanism for St. John's wort's antidepressant effect is unknown. It is standardized by percentage of hypericin, one of the active ingredients. But hypericin is not thought to be the ingredient responsible for the antidepressant effect (Bratman & Girman, 2003). Hyperforin, another component, may be responsible for the antidepressant effect. There is some evidence that it inhibits the reuptake of serotonin, GABA, and L-glutamate (Kuhn & Winston, 2000). Linde et al. (1996) noted that hypericum extracts have at least ten groups of components that may cause its pharmacological effects. More likely, it is the synergistic combination of ingredients. It does appear that St. John's wort relieves depression by preventing the reuptake of serotonin, the same mechanism as SSRIs (e.g., Prozac, Zoloft).

Some have speculated that St. John's wort's antidepressant effect could be due to its anti-inflammatory effect through the action of the flavonoids and flavonol glycosides (Kuhn & Winston, 2000). St. John's wort blocks the production of cytokines, the chemical messengers involved in inflammation (Balch, 2002). This link has not been reliably demonstrated, but it is intriguing given the discussion in Chapters 3 and 9 about the influence of cytokines on depression.

Some have expressed concern that St. John's wort functions as a monamine oxidase (MAO) inhibitor. It has been shown to function in this way in mice, but not in rats or humans (Bladt & Wagner, 1994; Bratman & Girman, 2003; Hale, 2004). As I describe in the next section, patients who take MAO inhibitors cannot eat or drink anything with tyramine, a substance found in aged foods. Yet St. John's wort is widely used in countries such as France without dietary restrictions, and people in these countries regularly consume cheese and red wine (both of which contain large amounts of tyramine).

Dosage

The standard dosage is 900 mg of St. John's wort per day (300 mg three times per day). It should be standardized to 0.3 percent hypericin. It generally takes four to six weeks to take effect (Bratman & Girman, 2003; Ernst, 2002; Kuhn & Winston, 2000). Combining St. John's wort with lemon balm increases its activity (Kuhn & Winston, 2000). It reaches peak level in the plasma in five hours, with a half-life of twenty-four to forty-eight hours.

Taken by itself, St. John's wort has an excellent safety record (Ernst, 2002). Herbalists often combine it with other herbs to address the range of symptoms that depressed people have (Kuhn & Winston, 2000). Some of these herbs incude schisandra, rosemary, black cohosh, and lavender.

Safety Concerns

Approximately 2.4 percent of patients who take St. John's wort develop side effects. The most common are mild stomach discomfort, allergic reactions, skin rashes, tiredness, and restlessness. Like other antidepressants, St. John's wort can trigger an episode of mania in vulnerable patients or patients with bipolar disorder (Bratman & Girman, 2003). St. John's wort can also cause photosensitivity.

Some of the more concerning safety issues have to do with drug interactions. St. John's wort accelerates the metabolism of several classes of medications, including anticonvulsants, cyclosporins, and birth control pills, leading to lower serum levels of the medication than prescribed (Ernst, 2002; Thomas Hale, personal communication, April 9, 2003). It can also interact with other serotonergic drugs, such as prescription antidepressants and can lead to serotonin syndrome (Bratman & Girman, 2003). Serotonin syndrome can be fatal, so prescription antidepressants should not be taken while taking St. John's wort (Harkness & Bratman, 2003). Since St. John's wort can interact with other medications, it is important for mothers to understand the need to inform their health care providers that they are taking the herb.

St. John's Wort and Breastfeeding

At this writing, the consensus appears to be that St. John's wort is safe for breastfeeding mothers. Hale (2004) lists St. John's wort as L2, "safer," meaning that no adverse effects in infants have been observed. Similarly, the *German Commission E Monographs* (Blumenthal et al., 1998), which lists the guidelines for use of herbs in Germany's national medical program, has listed St. John's wort as safe for both pregnancy and lactation. Finally, Humphrey (2003), in the *Nursing Mothers' Herbal,* gives St. John's wort a safety rating of B— "may not be appropriate for self-use by some individuals or dyads or may cause adverse effects if misused" (p. 272). She suggests that women who want to use St. John's wort seek reliable safety information.

Klier, Schafer, Schmid-Siegel, Lenz, and Mannel (2002) indicated that we still lack systematic information on the pharmacokinetics of St. John's wort in breast milk or infant plasma. In their case study, they examined four breast milk samples (including both fore and hind milk) from a mother taking the standard dose of St. John's wort (300 mg three times per day). They examined the samples for both hypericin and hyperforin. They found that only hyperforin was excreted into breast milk at a low level. Both hyperforin and hypericin were below the level of quantification in the infant's plasma. The authors recommended caution in prescribing this herb to breastfeeding mothers until long-term effects are clear.

When mothers ask about St. John's wort, it is important to inform them about these contradictory references and suggest that they discuss their options with their health care providers to determine the best approach. Age of the infant is another consideration, with younger infants being more vulnerable to exposure to medications. As Bratman and Girman (2003) noted, the maximum safe dosages for pregnant and lactating women have not yet been established, so some caution is wise.

Kava

Kava *(Piper methysticum)* has a long history of use in the Polynesian islands. Kava produces relaxation and is also believed to be antiseptic and anti-inflammatory. Its more common use is for anxiety, and it operates on the same receptors as the benzodiazepines (e.g., Xanax). Kavalactones (the active ingredient) also promote relaxation of the skeletal muscles. It is often mixed in preparations with St. John's wort to treat anxiety and depression, although some recommend that people with depression avoid kava (Kuhn & Winston, 2000). Some evidence shows that it is effective in reducing anxiety, nervousness, and tension without reducing alertness (Ernst, 2002). It has also been used for chronic pain conditions and sleep disorders (Kuhn & Winston, 2000).

Even with a long history of use in other cultures, some serious concerns about this herb have been raised. Although side effects are relatively rare (occurring in approximately 2 percent of patients), they are serious (Ernst, 2002). Kava interacts with other medications, including antidepressants, benzodiazepines, alcohol, and sleeping pills, and has potentially dangerous side effects including liver damage (usually with a high dose). The Food and Drug Administration has issued a consumer advisory. It is currently contraindicated for breastfeeding mothers (Balch, 2002; Hale, 2004; Kuhn & Winston, 2000). Even non-breastfeeding mothers should not try to self-medicate with this herb and should seek assistance from a licensed herbalist if they are interested in using it.

Summary

Mothers who are interested in trying herbs may find that St. John's wort is appropriate for them in treating depression. Numerous studies have found it as effective as standard antidepressants, and it appears to be safe for breastfeeding mothers. There is some concern about possible drug interactions.

At this time, kava is an herb most mothers should avoid because of safety concerns. If mothers want to take it, they should do so only under the guidance of a licensed herbalist, naturopath, or other health care professional who is knowledgeable about herbs.

ANTIDEPRESSANTS

Medications for depression are often the first line of treatment offered to patients in a health care setting. Antidepressants are generally necessary for the treatment of major depression but may be used for mild and moderate depression as well. Medications can be combined with other treatment modalities.

Some patients resist the idea of taking medications for depression. When helping mothers weigh their options, one factor to consider is the severity of their depression. A mother who is severely impaired (e.g., cannot get out of bed, cannot stop crying) will almost certainly need medications. On the other hand, a mother with mild to moderate depression might be more interested in other approaches. It is also important to consider the type of symptoms present. According to Preston and Johnson (2004), medications are especially helpful in treating the following symptoms: sleep disturbance, especially early-morning awakening or hypersomnia; appetite disturbance, eating too much or too little; fatigue; decreased sex drive; diurnal variations in mood (e.g., feeling worse in the morning); restlessness or agitation; impaired concentration; and pronounced anhedonia (the inability to experience pleasure). A mother with these symptoms is likely to benefit from medications. If depression is severe and/or patients have these types of symptoms, medications are probably the best approach.

Another aspect to assess is the mother's feelings about being on medications. If she is adamant that she does not want medications she is more likely to be noncompliant if she feels medications were forced upon her. In this case, assuming her depression is not severe, the alternative approaches in Chapters 9 and 10 may be more attractive to her. It can also be helpful to develop a treatment plan in which one approach, such as exercise, is tried for a certain number of weeks. If the depression has not improved, then medications can be tried. Or the health care provider might suggest a trial of medication for a certain number of weeks. If a mother knows that an endpoint is in sight, she may be more willing to try medication. This type of planning will make the mother an active participant in her own health care and will increase compliance.

There are three major types of antidepressants. All work to increase the amount of the neurotransmitters serotonin, norepinephrine, or dopamine available in the brain. The three categories are described in the following sections.

Tricyclics

Tricyclic antidepressants (TCAs) are the oldest and least expensive of the antidepressants. They have a solid track record of effectiveness and include medications such as Pamelor (nortriptyline) and Elavil (amitriptyline). They are effective but tend to have side effects that people do not like. Patient compliance is often a problem with TCAs. Once patients start to feel better, they may choose to discontinue the medications, and this can negatively affect their treatment. In one study, 41 percent of depressed patients stopped taking their medications at two weeks, and 68 percent had stopped by four weeks (Johnson, cited in Mynor-Wallis et al., 1995). Similarly, in a meta-analysis of sixty-two randomized trials, Anderson and Tomenson (1995) found that the discontinuation rate of medications was 10 percent lower for SSRIs than for TCAs, and that the study dropout rate due to side effects was 25 percent lower with the SSRIs.

TCAs have another serious drawback: the risk of suicide. Tricyclics can be lethal in too large a dose. If these medications are used, patients must be closely monitored and not given sufficient medication in each prescription period to provide the means to kill themselves. Preston and Johnson (2004) recommend the following medications as alternatives to TCAs for suicidal patients or those at high risk for suicide: fluoxetine (Prozac), sertraline (Zoloft), paroxetine (Paxil), or bupropion (Wellbutrin).

In one study, a TCA (nortriptyline) was used to prevent a recurrence of postpartum depression in women who had had a previous episode (Wisner et al., 2001). In this study, women who had had a previous episode were randomly assigned to receive either nortriptyline or a placebo. They received treatment immediately postpartum. At the end of the twenty-week treatment period, the same number of women in each group developed a recurrence (six in each group). The authors concluded that nortriptyline did not confer greater prevention than the placebo.

Tricyclics and Breastfeeding

Most tricyclics are compatible with breastfeeding. In a review of the literature, Wisner, Perel, and Findling (1996) found that tricyclic antidepressants appeared to have the best safety record in terms of accumulation of the medication in breast milk or quantifiable amounts in breastfeeding babies. The tricyclics they specifically named included amitriptyline, nortriptyline, desipramine, clomipramine, and dothiepin. They found that infants older than ten weeks are at lower risk for adverse effects, and there was no evidence of accumulation of these medications in infants. These medications, along with sertraline, were considered to be the treatments of choice for breastfeeding mothers. In contrast, doxepin and fluoxetine did have some adverse effects on infants, perhaps because they both have active metabolites (Hale, 2004).

Selective Serotonin Reuptake Inhibitors

SSRIs are the newest class of antidepressants, and include such well-known medications as fluoxetine (Prozac), sertraline (Zoloft), paroxetine (Paxil), and citalopram (Celexa). As their name implies, they work specifically on serotonin receptors. Although these medications still have side effects, they have fewer than the other antidepressants, and their dosing schedule is less complex. Many patients experience sexual side effects, particularly inorgasmia, and may stop taking their medications because of them. SSRIs are effective for approximately 80 percent of patients. If patients do not respond to one type of SSRI, another should be tried (Institute for Clinical Systems Improvement, 2004; Preston & Johnson, 2004). Even with their drawbacks, SSRIs work and can be a very effective tool in your arsenal of treatments for depression.

Because SSRIs have the potential for interacting with other medications, a careful history of other medications (prescription, over the counter, and herbal) should always be taken. SSRIs can be dangerous if taken with MAO inhibitors, nonsedating antihistamines (e.g., Hismanal), TCAs, and lithium because they may increase levels of each. Problems can also occur if they are taken with carbamazepine and St. John's wort (Preston & Johnson, 2004).

Venlafaxine (Effexor) was an effective treatment in a small, open-label study of fifteen women with major depression that developed within the first three months postpartum (Cohen et al., 2001). At the end of the eight-week trial, twelve of fifteen women experienced a remission of their depression.

SSRIs and Breastfeeding

SSRIs have also been studied with regard to breastfeeding. One study examined fluoxetine levels in nineteen breastfeeding women (Hendrick et al., 2001). Fluoxetine was present in 30 percent of the infant sera, and the fluoxetine metabolite norfluoxetine was present in 85 percent. Fluoxetine peaked in breast milk approximately eight hours after the mother's dose. A daily dose of 20 mg or less was significantly less likely to produce a detectable concentration than a dose that was higher than 20 mg per day. There were no adverse effects in any infants.

In a study of fourteen mother-infant breastfeeding pairs, Epperson and colleagues (2001) found that infants' exposure to sertraline during breastfeeding did not block platelet serotonin uptake in infants. This has relevance because serotonergic medications can have potentially harmful effects on babies' neurodevelopment. No infant in the study experienced adverse effects due to sertraline exposure. Indeed, levels of sertraline and its metabolite (desmethylsertraline) in the infants were at or below the lower limit of quantification.

Another study collected milk samples from ten mothers taking sertraline and blood samples from both the mothers and their babies. They found that the babies were receiving less than 2 percent of the mothers' dose (Dodd et al., 2000).

One case study of six mothers found that sertraline was associated with a decreased milk supply (Holland, 2000). The author was able to help mothers overcome this problem with increased oral fluids and by increasing the frequency of feeding.

In a study of two women who were taking fluvoxamine, Piontek, Wisner, Perel, and Peindl (2001) found that in each case, the drug was undetectable in the infants' sera. The drugs had no adverse effects during infancy, and the infants were healthy at two to three years of age.

Citalopram (Celexa) has been used in two studies. The first is a case study of a mother being treated for postpartum depression. When the mother's dose was 40 mg per day, the infant had detectable amounts of citalopram in the serum, and the infant's sleep was uneasy. When the mother's dose was reduced to 20 mg and two feedings were replaced with formula feedings, the infant's sleep normalized (Schmidt, Olesen, & Jensen, 2000). In another study of eleven mothers taking citalopram through pregnancy and lactation, the authors found that concentrations of the medications were two to three times higher in the milk than in the mother's plasma. But infant levels of citalopram and its metabolites were low or undetectable. Up until one year of age, neurodevelopment of these infants was normal. The authors noted that the infants had minimal exposure through lactation (Heikkinen, Ekblad, Kero, Ekblad, & Laine, 2002).

Paroxetine has also been studied with regard to breastfeeding. In this study, twenty-five sample sets were obtained from mother-infant pairs. All the mothers were taking paroxetine. The researchers found detectable levels of paroxetine in all maternal serum samples and twenty-four of twenty-five breast milk samples. However, in all the infant serum samples, paroxetine was below the lower limit of detection. There were no adverse effects in any infants. The mean infant dose of paroxetine was 1.1 percent of the maternal dose (Misri, Kim, Riggs, & Kostaras, 2000).

SSRIs are an effective treatment option for depression. Most are compatible with breastfeeding. There is some concern about Prozac and to a lesser extent Celexa because of their active metabolites and potential to expose infants to higher levels of the mother's dose (see Table 11.1). But they can be used if others are not effective.

MAO Inhibitors

MAO inhibitors are also very effective, but they have fallen out of favor because of the strict dietary restrictions associated with their use. MAO inhibitors include phenelzine (Nardil), isocarboxazid (Marplan), and tranylcypromine (Parnate). When taking these medications, patients cannot eat or drink anything containing tyramine. Tyramine is a byproduct of bacterial fermentation and is common in

TABLE 11.1. Safety of antidepressant medications for breastfeeding mothers.

Medication	Lactation risk category[a]	Theoretical infant dose[a]	Peak in mother's plasma[a,b]	Protein binding (%)[a,b]	Comments[a,b]
Fluoxetine (Prozac)	L2 for older infants; L3 for neonates	57 µg/kg per day	1.5-12 hours (peak at 6 hours)	94.5	Approved by American Academy of Pediatrics (AAP) for use during pregnancy. Active metabolites. Baby's intake 10-17 percent of mother's dose.
Paroxetine (Paxil)	L2	15.21 µg/kg per day	5-8 hours	95	Inactive metabolite. Preferable to Prozac.
Sertraline (Zoloft)	L2	21.45 µg/kg per day	7-8 hours	98	Metabolite (desmethylsertraline) is inactive. Preferable to Prozac.
Citalopram (Celexa)	L3	14.6 µg/kg per day	2-4 hours	80	Active metabolite. Baby's intake may be 3-4 percent of maternal dose.
Bupropion (Wellbutrin)	L3	28.4 µg/kg per day	2 hours	75-88	May concentrate in human milk. However, plasma levels of the drug were undetectable in the infant in one case study.

TABLE 11.1 *(continued)*

Medication	Lactation risk category[a]	Theoretical infant dose[a]	Peak in mother's plasma[a,b]	Protein binding (%)[a,b]	Comments[a,b]
Amitriptyline (Elavil)	L2	21.4 µg/kg per day	2-4 hours	94.8	Estimated that the nursing infant would receive less than 1 percent of maternal dose.
Imipramine (Tofranil)	L2	4.35 µg/kg per day	1-2 hours	90	Could accumulate in infant plasma, although it has not been reported. Infant should be monitored closely.
Nortriptyline (Pamelor)	L2	27.0 µg/kg per day	7-8.5 hours	92	In one case study, the relative dose in milk was 2.3 percent of the maternal dose. However, others have not been able to detect it in maternal milk or infant serum.

Sources: [a]Hale, T.W. (2004). *Medications and mothers' milk.* Amarillo, TX: Pharmasoft. Used with permission; [b]Lawrence, R. & Lawrence, T. (1999). *Breastfeeding: A guide for the medical profession.* St. Louis: Mosby.

L2 = "safer"—risk is remote; L3 = "moderately safe"—given only if potential benefit justifies potential risk to the infant.

foods such as red wine and cheese. When these foods are consumed with an MAO inhibitor, hypertensive crisis or even death can occur. They are not widely used in the United States but may be prescribed if other medications have failed. They are also effective in the treatment of atypical depression (Institute for Clinical Systems Improvement, 2004). These medications are enjoying a renaissance of use, however, because if the dietary restrictions are observed, some feel they are safer than tricyclics and have fewer side effects (Preston & Johnson, 2004).

The MAO inhibitors are not included in Table 11.1. According to Hale (personal communication, September 9, 2003), these medications are not safe for breastfeeding mothers. There is some concern that the medications may cause a permanent change or destroy the baby's ability to produce MAO, and the risk does not outweigh the benefits.

Deciding on an Antidepressant

Making a decision about which antidepressant to use can be complex. But some guidelines exist that can help narrow the decision. Remick (2002) recommended the following considerations. First, has the patient been on a particular antidepressant before and did she have a positive response to it? Second, if a patient is possibly suicidal, a tricyclic or MAO inhibitor would not be a good choice since these medications are potentially lethal in overdose or in combination with certain foods. The side effect profile of the antidepressants should also be considered. These side effects include sedation, weight gain, orthostatic hypotension, and sexual dysfunction, and can be more or less troubling for individual patients. Another consideration is other medications a patient is currently taking; possible drug-drug interactions should also guide the choice. Finally, costs need to be considered. The newer SSRIs are considerably more expensive than the older tricyclics and MAO inhibitors. For patients without drug coverage, this can be a deciding factor.

Wisner et al. (1996) recommended that mothers be actively involved in the decision about whether to use medications. It is important to respect a mother's wish to continue breastfeeding. Wisner et al. recommended that mothers and fathers be included in the discussion of risks and benefits associated with breastfeeding with medications, not breastfeeding, and being raised by a chronically depressed mother. Before medication starts, mothers and their doctors should observe the infant for alertness, activity, sleep, and feeding patterns. They also advised that serum levels of infants less than ten weeks old be measured once mothers have settled on their minimum effective dose. In infants older than ten weeks, the serum levels should be measured only if there are behavior changes from baseline. Wisner et al. recommended charting any discussion of medications with mothers, as well as discussions about weaning, attempting nondrug treatments, and the mother's competence to consent to treatment.

Medications and Breastfeeding

In considering which medications are most compatible with breastfeeding, the factors to consider are when the medication peaks in concentration in the mother's blood, protein binding, and the nature of the metabolites (Hale, 2004; Lawrence & Lawrence, 1999). Table 11.1 lists these factors and the lactation risk category for the tricyclic and SSRI classes of antidepressants. The newest SSRI, Lexapro, is a metabolite of Celexa, so the same classifications apply to it (Hale, 2004).

Peak. This is the time it takes from the administration of the drug to the point at which the level of medication is highest in the mother's plasma. For example, a medication may reach peaks in a mother's plasma six hours after she takes it, so she should avoid breastfeeding at six hours. Mothers should avoid breastfeeding during the peak. But they not need to pump and dump their milk because the medications are reabsorbed by the body and exit the milk compartment as plasma levels of the medication fall (Hale, 2004). (Some medications, such as barbiturates and iodides, can become trapped in the milk and will need to be discarded, however.)

Protein binding. Drugs circulate bound to maternal plasma albumin. The higher the percentage of protein binding, the less likely this medication is to enter the milk. Good protein binding is greater than 90 percent (Hale, 2004).

Metabolites. The metabolites are the component parts of a medication as it breaks down during digestion. Medications with active metabolites dramatically increase the baby's exposure to the medication.

For example, Prozac has active metabolites, so the baby receives 10 to 17 percent of the maternal dose. In contrast, Zoloft has inert metabolites, and the baby receives less than 1 percent of the mother's dose (Hale, 2004; Lawrence & Lawrence, 1999).

MEDICATIONS FOR COMORBID CONDITIONS

As I described in Chapter 1, there is now increased awareness of the presence of conditions comorbid with postpartum depression. If a condition is co-occurring with postpartum depression, the woman may need medications for it as well. I do not attempt to list every medication that is useful in treating these conditions, but only the more common ones and those most likely to be prescribed.

Chronic Pain

Two major classes of antidepressants are effective in pain management: TCAs and SSRIs. Of these, Elavil is the most effective for the treatment of pain, but it also is the most sedating and has the most side effects. Pamelor and Norpramin have fewer side effects but are also less effective (Schneider, 2001). Tricyclics in dosages between 75 and 200 mg per day can be expected to relieve pain in 55 to 67 percent of patients (Marcus, 2000).

The SSRIs can also be used for chronic pain. Some patients become agitated on these medications, and they can cause insomnia. On the other hand, for patients with overwhelming fatigue, these medications can provide a needed boost. This class includes fluoxetine (Prozac), sertraline (Zoloft), paroxetine (Paxil), and citalopram (Celexa).

Generally, for the treatment of chronic pain, tricyclics are better than SSRIs (Schneider, 2001). In terms of breastfeeding, the recommendations are the same as in the previous section. Table 11.1 lists which antidepressants are most compatible with breastfeeding.

PTSD

Several classes of medications are used to treat PTSD. Antidepressants are the most common, but adrenergic agents, serotonin-2 antagonists/reuptake inhibitors (SARIs), and anticonvulsants are also used.

Antidepressants

Antidepressants are a key part of treatment of PTSD in that they address PTSD symptoms and comorbid depression. The SSRIs appear to be the most effective, but other types can also be helpful.

SSRIs address all three classes of symptoms: intrusive thoughts, avoidance and numbing, and hyperarousal (Friedman, 2001). Of the SSRIs, fluoxetine (Prozac) and sertraline (Zoloft) have been most successful, although higher doses may be required for PTSD than for depression (Preston & Johnson, 2004). Some of the side effects associated with SSRIs can be managed with the addition of other medications to the regimen. A common class of medication that gets combined with SSRIs are the SARIs.

Serotonin-2 Antagonists/Reuptake Inhibitors

Trazodone (Desyrel) and nefazodone (Serzone) are SARIs, which, when administered alongside an SSRI, boost the actions of these drugs and reverse medication-induced insomnia. Both trazodone and nefazodone are sedative and may be taken at bedtime (Bezchilibnzyk-Butler & Jeffries, 1999). Trazodone suppresses REM sleep. This acts to reduce the number of nightmares patients experience (Lange, Lange, & Cabaltica, 2000). In contrast, nefazodone increases REM sleep and improves overall sleep quality (Bezchilibnzyk-Butler & Jeffries, 1999). Both of these drugs may be too sedating for some patients, however (Friedman, 2001).

In terms of breastfeeding, trazodone appears to be the better choice. The percentage of the maternal dose that the infant is exposed to is 0.6 percent (Hale, 2004). In contrast, nefezodone has active metabolites. Hale (2004) states, "this medication should probably not be used in breastfeeding mothers with young infants, premature infants, infants subject to apnea, or other weakened infants" (p. 592).

Adrenergic Agents

Another class of medications used with PTSD is the adrenergic agents. They work by blocking norepinephrine receptors and include clonidine (Catapres) and guanfacine (Tenex). Propranolol (Inderal) is also used, but not when a patient has comorbid depression (Friedman, 2001). Adrenergic agents are frequently prescribed to control hypertension, but in patients with PTSD, they also control symptoms of intrusive memories and hyperarousal.

Clonidine is excreted into human milk, with the baby receiving about 6.8 percent of the mother's dose. It may also reduce prolactin, which can influence milk production early postpartum. Guanfacine has not been studied with regard to human milk. However, Hale (2004) notes that since this medication has low molecular weight, a high volume of distribution, and penetrates the central nervous system, it is likely to penetrate the milk. Both of these medications are rated L3, "moderately safe," for use only if potential benefit outweighs the potential risk to the infant (Hale, 2004).

Anticonvulsants

Anticonvulsants are another category of medications used in the treatment of PTSD. The two most commonly used are carbamazepine (Tegretol) and valproate (Depakote). Both are effective in managing symptoms of bipolar disorder, but also help with PTSD symptoms. Carbamazepine is effective for intrusive memories and hyperarousal, and valproate helps with avoidance, numbing, and hyperarousal (Friedman, 2001).

Carbamazepine's side effects include drowsiness, headache, dizziness, weight gain, adverse hematologic effects (including aplastic anemia and leukopenia), and lower thyroxine levels. Carbamazepine has been approved by the American Academy of Pediatrics for use in breastfeeding mothers. Very little appears in the breast milk or in breastfeeding infants. It peaks in the breast milk four to five hours after the medication is taken (Hale, 2004).

Valproate also has side effects including weight gain, elevation of hepatic transaminase levels, and menstrual disturbances. It is contraindicated in patients with liver dysfunction. This medication has also been approved by the American Academy of Pediatrics for use in breastfeeding mothers. Hale (2004) notes that it is most likely safe, but recommends that the infant be monitored for liver and platelet changes.

Bipolar Disorder

Some of the medications used for PTSD are also used for bipolar disorder. These include carbamazepine and valproate. The data that exist in terms of breastfeeding and these medications is somewhat scarce. Generally, both are considered compatible with breastfeeding, although some levels of toxicity have been reported.

Carbamazepine

In a review, Chaudron and Jefferson (2000) found fifty cases of carbamazepine use during breastfeeding. Only ten of these cases reported on infant serum levels, and two noted infant hepatic dysfunction. As noted, it has been approved by the American Academy of Pediatrics for use in breastfeeding mothers (Hale, 2004).

Valproate

Similarly, Chaudron and Jefferson (2000) found thirty-nine cases of valproate use during breastfeeding, eight of which reported infant serum levels. Of these infants, there was one case of thrombocytopenia and one case of anemia. This medication has also been approved by the American Academy of Pediatrics for use in breastfeeding mothers. Hale (2004) notes that it is most likely safe, but recommends that the infant be monitored for liver and platelet changes.

In another study of six breastfeeding pairs, none of the women had taken valproate during pregnancy, but all started taking it postpartum to prevent a recurrence of bipolar disorder (Piontek, Baab, Peindl, & Wisner, 2000). The infants' blood levels were 0.9 to 2.3 percent of the maternal dose. These levels were lower than has been reported in previous studies. Four of the six infants were under four weeks of age when the study began. This study is unique because it can determine levels strictly from breastfeeding rather than exposure during pregnancy.

Lithium

In the case of lithium, opinion has changed in recent years. It used to be that lithium was always contraindicated for breastfeeding mothers. But Chaudron and Jefferson (2000) noted that a change might be in order. They found eleven cases in the literature of lithium use during breastfeeding, eight of which reported infant serum levels, and two reported symptoms consistent with infant toxicity. They concluded that a woman's historic response to a medication should be the prime consideration in selecting it rather than rejecting medications outright.

The American Academy of Pediatrics has urged caution when using lithium in breastfeeding mothers. Since lithium can accumulate in the baby, the baby's lithium levels must be closely monitored. Lithium can also affect the infant's production of thyroxine, so the baby's thyroid levels should be monitored as well. The medication takes ten days to reach a steady state in the mother, so the infant's lithium levels should be monitored after that, unless the infant is showing symptoms of lithium toxicity (e.g., infant is floppy, unresponsive, and has inverted T waves). Although this medication is not automatically contraindicated, carbamazepine or valproate may be safer choices (Hale, 2004).

PHASES OF DEPRESSION MANAGEMENT WITH MEDICATION

In this section, I discuss depression management with medication. Such management has three main phases: acute, continuation, and maintenance (Lesperance & Frasure-Smith, 2000). Knowing about the phases of management can help you communicate a treatment plan more effectively to mothers.

Acute Phase

The acute phase occurs during the first six to twelve weeks of the depressive episode. This begins with the first dose and lasts until the patient is asymptomatic (Preston & Johnson, 2004). The objectives during this stage are to rapidly reduce symptoms of depression and to monitor patients for the risk of suicide. It is important to evaluate whether the antidepressant you prescribed is effective. If it is not, there are two possible explanations: the dose is inadequate, or treatment has not been sufficiently lengthy for an adequate response (Institute for Clinical Systems Improvement, 2004). Assessments should include an evaluation of symptoms, work or school productivity, and whether interpersonal relationships have improved.

In this phase, it is also important to talk to patients about what they should expect from medications. Patients who are adequately educated are more likely to comply with treatments when they understand side effects and have realistic expectations about what medications will do. Preston and Johnson (2004) recommend that the following be part of educating patients about medication use:

1. Medications may take ten to twenty-one days before patients notice a difference in symptoms.
2. When symptoms do improve, it is likely that they will be the ones with a biological basis, such as sleep disturbance. They may not help with more psychologically based symptoms such as self-esteem.
3. Treatment is working when patients are sleeping better, have less daytime fatigue, and have some improvement in emotional control.
4. There may be side effects, but these can be managed.
5. The total length of time to be on antidepressants varies for each individual.
6. Antidepressants are not addictive.

Continuation Phase

The continuation phase lasts from four to nine months. The objective during this phase is to prevent a relapse of symptoms, which can occur if treatment is terminated during this time (Lesperance & Frasure-Smith, 2000). If symptoms have not improved, or if the patient has relapsed, it is appropriate to reevaluate both the diagnosis and patient compliance. Are there comorbid conditions (especially substance abuse) that are keeping treatments from being effective? Is the medication effective for the patient or should another be tried? Is the patient complying with treatment and taking the medications at the appropriate intervals?

A larger dose may be needed in some cases, or the patient may need to be on the medication for a longer period of time. Preston and Johnson (2005) noted that the most common mistake that family physicians make is to undermedicate their depressed patients. Generally, the length of an adequate trial is four to six weeks. If the medication is not effective after that time, another medication should be considered. Or an additional medication could be added to the regimen (Institute for Clinical Systems Improvement, 2004).

Maintenance Phase

This phase should be initiated for patients who have had multiple episodes of depression, who have particularly severe or difficult-to-treat episodes, and are therefore at high risk of recurrence. This phase may be for life in some patients, particularly those who have had multiple episodes of major depression.

CONCLUSION

Both conventional and herbal antidepressants offer hope to women with postpartum depression and related conditions. These medications can treat even severe depression, and most are compatible with breastfeeding. These treatments can be combined with other modalities described in the previous two chapters to give mothers additional tools to cope with future life stresses and increase their sense of competence and self-efficacy.

Chapter 12

Postpartum Depression and Psychosis: One Woman's Story

When I was working on the first edition of this book, a young woman named Jenny contacted me. She told me that she had suffered from postpartum depression and psychosis in the recent past and was anxious to share her story for the benefit of other mothers. What made Jenny's story absolutely unique was that she had kept a diary before and during her experience and as she recovered.

She has shared her diary with me, as well as the medical records from the state hospital. They provide a fascinating glimpse inside postpartum mental illness. This story was so compelling, I wanted to include it in this edition as well.

When preparing to write this edition, I contacted her again. Eleven years had elapsed since our first contact. During that time, she has had four more children with no recurrence of postpartum psychosis or depression. She has also published her own full-length account of her experiences. It is available at <www.naturalfamilyco.com>.

BACKGROUND

Jenny relates her illness to a number of different factors. Jenny feels she was vulnerable to postpartum illness because of her health history and her lifelong struggle with severe allergies. In addition to her health history, she experienced a series of stressors in both the pre- and postpartum periods, which are described later. In the years that have elapsed since our first contact, she has also recovered memories of two previous sexual assaults: one during childhood, the second during her hospitalization. She has added this information to her account.

Jenny was twenty years old when she had her first child. Her marriage and the birth of her daughter within less than a year constituted two major life changes within a relatively short span of time. Nevertheless, she was happy with her new life and joyfully celebrated the birth of her first child. She was also buffered from the potential negative effects of these stressors by a large and supportive family, a close relationship with her parents, and strong religious faith.

Michelle H. was born exactly 76 hours ago. December 1, 1988, at 10:44 p.m. This will be a landmark day in my life. I was so overjoyed and emotionally ready for her to be here, and now she's here. . . . [My husband], Mom, Dad, and my sister and her husband were all there. It was an awesome moment.

As thrilled as she was with the birth of her daughter, her birth experience was stressful. Jenny does not feel that it was the sole or even main cause of her illness. Rather, it was the first link in a chain of events that led to her illness.

THE BIRTH EXPERIENCE

Jenny was very involved in the care she received during her pregnancy. Before the baby was born, she carefully prepared herself for labor and delivery, read extensively, exercised, and did yoga. Three weeks before her due date, she read two books on the Bradley method of natural childbirth. Although she had always wanted to have natural childbirth, these were the first books she had read that articulated what she wanted. Unfortunately, the hospital where she was to deliver specialized in high-risk patients and tended to intervene frequently, even in routine births—the hospital's rate of cesarean births was an alarming 50 percent. Since it was so close to her due date, she had no choice but to proceed with her doctor and the hospital. Even after making the decision to proceed, she knew it would be difficult to have a natural delivery in that setting.

My alarm grew as the week progressed. [My husband] and I went on a tour of [the hospital] and I freaked out. I had done everything backward. I chose my doctor then the hospital, then three weeks before giving birth, I discovered the method I wanted to use. Not exactly ideal. According to Bradley, you choose the facility, then the doctor and you know the method before you get pregnant. Anyway, the past four weeks have been hell as I've tried to convince [my husband], my doctor, my mom, and mostly myself that this was the method I wanted to use. At one point, I seriously considered changing doctor/hospital but we recognized that most doctors won't take on a patient this late in the game.

Knowing I'd have a fight on my hands, I read the Bradley Method three times to fully acquaint myself with the techniques—(all relaxation, deep breathing, concentration) and all the arguments for not having "procedures" done at the hospital, to me or the baby.

During her lengthy labor (more than twenty-four hours), one of the more negative aspects was the way she describes being treated by the hospital staff. At one point, she was alone in a hospital room on a table. She had only a sheet over her, and she was very cold. An intern, who was apparently inexperienced, came in and gave her a rough and lengthy examination. Another doctor examined her, then the intern and the other doctor discussed Jenny's progress with each other in front of her.

. . . then I began having a hard contraction. She [the second doctor] put her hands on my abdomen and instructed the intern to do likewise. They both were pushing and poking. I about lost control. I realized that he was the teachee and she was the teacher and I was the guinea pig. When my contraction was over I said "don't ever touch me while I'm having a contraction again."

At this point, Jenny asked to see her husband, who had been outside the room talking to her doctor on the telephone.

When I saw [my husband] I almost started to cry. I had asked three nurses for a blanket because I was frozen. I was cold, hurting and those dumb doctors had been using my laboring body to teach each other what a contraction should feel like.

Jenny and her husband were given the option of going home, walking, or being admitted to a labor room. She could not be admitted to the birthing room, as she requested, because she was only 2 to 3 cm dilated. They decided to go home. The Bradley method states that solitude, quiet, physical comfort, and physical relaxation are essential for the laboring woman. During the hours at the hospital, none of these were available. She labored at home for the next few hours and started to make progress. She arrived at the hospital again, hoping to go directly to the birthing room after being checked at her doctor's office.

When we arrived at the hospital, I was cold, tense, and nervous that I would get a lot of crap from the hospital staff. I sat in a wheelchair during *nine* contractions. As usual, they had miscommunicated the doctor's request for me. One nurse said I had to go to triage to "get checked." Another said I couldn't drink anything when she saw me take a sip of Vernors pop. Another said the birthing room wasn't prepped. (We had called 1/2 hour before from the clinic to tell them we were on our way.) No time to prep? Bull! I sat in that wheelchair getting madder and madder. Finally, I asked the admitting nurse if I could go labor in a labor bed until I was ready because I was having a hard time controlling my contractions. She called the birthing room to ask. They said "No, we're just about done." I had *two* more contractions while they finished. I was almost crying by now. I kept thinking of how wonderful I had felt at home, the contractions didn't even hurt while I was in the shower with the hot air *[sic]* beating on my back.

She sat in the lobby of the hospital in a wheelchair for thirty minutes while in active labor. Once she got into the birthing room, she continued to have trouble with the hospital staff over the issue of continuous fetal monitoring. Prior to coming back to the hospital, her doctor had agreed to intermittent fetal monitoring (ten minutes every hour), but the nurses kept insisting that she have continuous fetal monitoring. At one point, they even threatened to make her leave if she did not comply. When she was 5 cm dilated, her doctor ruptured her membranes. Three hours later, her daughter was born. In spite of the difficulties, it was a joyous occasion.

THE POSTPARTUM PERIOD

Approximately eight weeks after her daughter was born, Jenny and her husband moved to another state. This pulled Jenny away from her support network, including her close-knit family. During this time, her husband's back went out, adding to the stress of their move, as he was unable to help with either child care or the move. Nevertheless, Jenny was happy in her new role and enjoyed their new home.

It's so wonderful to be a mother. I've dreamed and planned to be one all my life. [My daughter] is everything to me, besides [my husband], and I would die for her. She's pretty and personable and I'm flattered that she wants to be with me most. It makes me feel good to see that satisfied look on her little face when she's done eating and I love to think that her little body is receiving nourishment and growth from my body.

Within approximately six weeks of their move to another state, Jenny developed postpartum psychosis. During the weeks prior to her psychosis, she had read a book about allergies that listed a number of food and environmental allergens. This book recommended a five-day fast as a way of locating allergy-producing substances. Having suffered from allergies all her life, she took this very seriously. She started to fast, even though she was breastfeeding, in an attempt to locate the foods and substances that caused allergic reactions. She was also getting fewer and fewer hours of sleep each night, insisting she could handle everything. As the days went by, she became increasingly manic. In this state, she took everything to its extreme, including trying to purify her body and her household environment by getting rid of all plastic and turning off her heat because there was a natural gas leak in her home. Here is her retrospective description of what happened to her. She wrote this account shortly after she was released from the psychiatric hospital.

It started slowly, then built to a peak. I became paranoid about being clean, purity, being perfect. I wanted to be a savior: save the town, the ward, the state, everyone. I wanted the millennium to start. I wanted to go to the temple to see Christ face to face. I wanted to live the word of wisdom perfectly. I cut out sugar, chocolate, meat, and ate only whole organic foods. I fasted. [My baby] looked hungry when my mom arrived. I kept freaking out, thinking [my husband] was going to die, someone was going to kill me, steal [my baby], etc. . . . It was hell!

I sang hymns all the time to ward off evil thoughts and spirits. I ran to Main Street, staying in the light, cast Satan out of [town], took my clothes off to my garments, sat down in the Lotus position looking at the sun, and waited. A police woman came up and tried to talk to me. She called [my husband]. He came and tried to get me to come home. They threw me in the ambulance and I came to. I put on my clothes, declared I was fine, and did my banking. [My husband] flipped out. He called the bishop, and my parents. I asked my mom to come down.

Her parents and husband took her to the hospital where she had delivered, but she refused to check herself in. From there, she went to the state hospital for nine days in her parents' state, then a private hospital for nine days, then back to the state hospital for six days, and finally back to the private hospital for two weeks. After her release, she convalesced at her parents' home for one month before returning home with her husband.

THE HOSPITAL DIARY

The next section of Jenny's story is taken from the diary she kept while in the state and private mental hospitals (the first time at each one). She wrote this account while she was hospitalized for post-partum psychosis. Much of the journal is dedicated to trying to make sense of what had happened to her.

March 29, 1989 This is going to be the most important journal I've ever kept. I'm in a mental hospital, [name of state hospital]. On Friday, I'm moving to a new hospital, [name of private hospital]. I'm confused though. Talking helps. I'm hoping this journal will help. I asked mom to bring it to me. Everyone here is very nice. They are all trying to help me get better.

March 30, 1989, 7:19 a.m. I woke up this morning and my breasts were aching (forced weaning). I asked the nurse for some Tylenol. She brought me some and I feel better. I exercised, prayed, watched the news, ate a banana that Mom gave me yesterday (day before yesterday), and I feel good. . . . I cried this morning because I miss [my baby]. I want to nurse her so bad but I've accepted that I won't be able to ever again—that hurts. I loved to think that it was my body that helped to make her grow. What a lift! But I can deal with it. I miss her smilin' face.

7:43 a.m. I've been thinking of an analogy to what has happened. It goes like this. Imagine yourself getting kicked in the head. But there is no tissue damage, no blood, no bruise, only your brain has been hurt. The hurt is very bad and you try to make it better but don't know what to do. You scream and cry and try to hurt yourself. You act totally irrational. As time goes by, the hurt starts to heal, somehow. The cells repair themselves (analogy), the tissue rebuilds, all that is really needed is some time, rest, good food, a listening ear and a notebook with a pen. The memory comes back and with it dark images, so evil, and bad that you cry, but also light, God, hope, love and peace. These images fight each other for space in your conscious. As time goes by, the light is the one that prevails and sanity or at least peace is restored. The dark images return sometimes to scare and frighten but eventually the light prevails and everything is OK. Now, I just need time to understand why and sort things out. It hurts to think I went through so much. Sometimes I'm embarrassed by my behavior. I want to crawl under a rock. But I'm also relieved because so much that was unexplainable is now understood.
. . . I'm still not myself. I have so many questions. And every time I ask one of the patients, they either look at me crazy or they give me their philosophy on life. The nurses try to answer my questions, but they are very busy and the doctors are great but they have even less time and many demands. It's OK, Mom said [private hospital] will be much better and they'll answer my questions and clear up any confusions. I can't wait to go. I just know it's *got* to

be better than this place. I don't hate it here, but I can see that it's holding me back from getting better.

8:55 a.m. I can't help having the feeling that the nurses and everyone keep lying to me and there is some major plot against me. They tell me one thing, then do another. They told me the gynecologist would be here at 8:30. Well, it's long past. They don't understand that to me a minute is like an hour and a day is like a month. Even five minutes seems like a year. Time is relative I know, but I wish they would tell the truth. I'm so confused as it is.

. . . I wish they'd come soon. I don't want them to take any blood. I hope they don't. I really am afraid to go see these doctors. I don't know them and they are going to touch the most private parts of my body. I usually don't have a problem with this, but now I'm scared. It's weird how you can change so quickly. I still am confused. I want answers *now!!*

12:10 p.m. I finally saw the doctors at 9:30 a.m. It's so hard to *wait!* They were cool. Wanted to take some blood but I said "no." Wanted to do a pelvic, I said "no way." I'm feeling too vulnerable right now. I need some time before they do these things again. I still think I'm going to refuse drugs at any cost. I'm having a hard enough time getting control and I really think what I need is some sleep.

I would say 95% of this problem is physical. The doctors and everyone keep talking about "chemical" but I think sleep deprivation is a real disease and I haven't had "good" sleep in *so long.* And the food changes that I imposed upon myself were a large part of this too so I understand why—at least some of the whys, but I still have quite a few to figure out. I have a lot of questions, but each second something new comes to me. The greatest thing is the way [my husband] and the family are supporting me. They are the greatest in the world. They have been visiting, bringing me food, talking on the phone and in person. They don't realize how much that helps. For four days, I was in isolation. I didn't know where I was, what was going on or where any of my family were, and I was scared to death. So scared, hurt, afraid, lonely, I wanted to die, that was *all* that I wanted.

About 10 times during the isolation, I thought OK, this is it, here I go, and then something would happen and I would be released for another few minutes, hours, seconds until the next death wish came. It peaked on Saturday night when I wanted to die for the last time. My tongue was lolling around in my head, I was dazed and confused. I hurt all over, my body was convulsing but all I wanted to do was die. The doctor was truly hurting my arm with the I.V. and instead of dying, I fell asleep. It was so depressing. When I woke up on Easter Sunday, I couldn't understand why I was alive. I didn't know what Christ wanted me to do. I had done everything I could to purify my life and body and he still didn't want to see me face to face.

[After receiving a blessing that night from my father, the death wishes stopped.] . . . Then I became suspicious of everyone. I thought they were trying to poison me with the food. I thought they were draculas taking my blood. I pulled out the I.V. and the catheter because I *knew* God wanted me to do it.

March 31, 1989 8:00 a.m. Today has finally arrived! I get to leave this pit of despair. *Everyone* is so pathetic here. . . . I was *so* angry last night. I kept imagining doing terrible things. The thing is I'm a good person. I want to do what's right. I have a daughter who needs me, a husband who needs me, and I don't need to be in this shit-hole prison. So why the hell am I here?????? I didn't commit any crime and I practically have to ask permission to pee. They try to poison me with this shit they call food and surround me with so much smoke it's like a bar. I hate it *here*. . . . I keep seeing myself in [town name], singing hymns, and casting out Satan. The policewoman came up to me and asked me to get dressed. Poor lady. As I was sitting there in the full Lotus position with my hands in the symbol of knowledge pose, all I can remember is this guy walking by and saying to her "This isn't exactly Mr. Rodger's [sic] neighborhood, is it?" And me, wanting to laugh but knowing I couldn't because it was too solemn a moment, and Satan would get my soul if I moved before [my husband] got there. Then he arrived and said, "Jenn, you've gotta come home," and I did, but I was *very* sick.

At this point, she was transferred to the private mental hospital. The following are excerpts taken from her diary written during that time.

March 31, 5:00 p.m. I'm finally here. It's nice. I'm exhausted. The orientation helped. I have so many questions but mostly I want to rest. I feel nervous, tense, overwhelmed. I had an in-tense *[sic]* evaluation, a medical check-up, an evaluation with a shrink (he was nice, not Dr. S., but a good guy). . . .

April "Fools" Day, 1989. Just met with Dr. S. He's an ass. Really. Wants me to take drugs. I just kept saying "nope." He can't force me unless I have another psychotic episode. I'm going to do everything I can to avoid that. But I *refuse* to fall into their mode of medicate, medicate, medicate. All I need is some sleep, some good food, and a chance to get my wits about me. . . . He kept tryin' to say I needed drugs. He doesn't know a damn thing about me except that I did some outrageous things out of the norm.

. . . I'm not just going to roll with it folks. I'm going to fight them *every* step of the way and I'm going to question *everything*. Sorry if that's in-con-*VIEN*-ient, but it's the way it goes. I'm going to get along with everyone and get the hell out of here.

Later. This place is awful. What I was just thinking is if it is such a great place and does so much good, why the hell has my roommate been here *six* times? . . . She is *so* doped up and screwed in the head by all the probing, searching to find out why, that I think she's on the verge of suicide. Well, she told me she was. Everyone here seems doped up, suicidal and depressed.

. . . I think this *all* could have been avoided *if* Mom and Dad had taken me home, put me to bed and let me sleep it off. But I was in a psychotic state when they showed up and I know they were scared by my behavior. So, like everyone else, take her to DRS. GOD. *They* will make everything better. Bullshit! All they did was scare the shit out of me and isolate me from my family.

This place is the same. They have buckets of pills, lots of analysis and isolation. *Most* of the people here need these things because they are suicidal. I am *not* suicidal. I'm just a tired Mom who was put in a situation [new home town] that was hard to handle and freaked out. I had too too too much pressure. No sleep (for a month) and I changed my eating habits. Those things plus all the pressure of the move, my callings, [my husband's] calling, Bradley Method of childbirth classes, fear of Satanism in [new town], pressure to be the best wife, best mother, best friend, best ward member, best sister, best daughter, best actress, best children's theater director, best temple-goer, cleanest house, cleanest healthiest body, cleanest healthiest well-behaved baby, best body, best reader, best student, best sister-in-law, best daughter-in-law, best gardener, best reader, most intelligent church-goer, best talker, best listener, best EVERYTHING, was *too* much. I need a vacation. That's what [hospital] is to me. I'm going to sleep, read, eat, and write—journal, letters, and I'm not going to listen to my doctor too much.

. . . I'm very suspicious of a doctor who doesn't even know me coming in and telling me I "need" drugs to make me "feel good." Sorry, that just doesn't cut it. If he said "you have an infection, I want you to help it get better," I'd take them. But I *don't* believe in "feel good" drugs and dammit *nobody* is going to make me take them. I'm not going to become one of "these" zombies who walk around pretending everything is fine. I know that I have a problem. I want to know what caused it, what I can do to avoid it in the future, and how I can get better.

April 1st, 7:40 p.m. Well, it's been a helluva day. I've been harassed by just about everybody to take the drugs (yes, including [my husband] and Mom). . . . [After a discussion with her doctor] he began pushing the drugs earnestly. He even tried to "bargain" with me. "I'll let you see your baby if you take the medicine." Nope. Those types of statements make me so curious to know *why* he feels the drugs are so important. I am *convinced* that the psychosis I experienced in [state name] was worst when I had no sleep, was eating little or fasting and when I was really tired. Nobody else seems to be. . . . I admit I have a problem. I want to get better and I want to know why but I *have* to do it *my* way. This is just like the birth. Hopefully, they'll understand.

THE PSYCHIATRIC EVALUATION

During the time that this diary was written, the doctors at the mental hospitals were keeping their own records. The following are excerpts from these records that describe Jenny's illness from the medical perspective. The first entries were made at the time Jenny was discharged from the state hospital to the private hospital. Following are excerpts from the combined psychiatric examination and summary note.

Mental status: This is a 21 year old, white female who appears to be her stated age. She is of moderate build. The patient is very agitated and disoriented. Her affect is blunted. Her mood went from hostile to tearful and scared. The patient denied being depressed but stated that she was very tired. The patient denied any suicidal or homicidal thoughts. She was preoccupied with religious grandiose delusions, stating "I was chosen by Jesus to fill a mission on this earth. I don't need a doctor. Jesus will heal me. I will fast until he comes to heal me." The patient is oriented to person and time. The patient seems to be confused regarding the events of the last four or five days. The patient's long-term memory appears to be intact. Her judgment and insight are poor.

Clinical course and treatment in the hospital: The patient was admitted on 3/23/89 from [other hospital] on a Medical Certificate. The patient was admitted with four-point restraints due to her being uncooperative to admission procedures. She was nonverbal and her behavior was unpredictable. The patient was put into seclusion. She was refusing meals and drank five, eight ounce glasses of water. On 3/24/89 the patient remained in seclusion. She was very agitated and delusional. She received 2.5 mg of Haldol and refused to talk to the doctor and refused to take a shower or use the bathroom. On 3/25/89, the patient continued to be hostile, refused to put clothes on, or to eat or drink. The patient voided on the floor, refusing to use the bathroom. Haldol was given to the patient. She received Benadryl 25 mg due to a dystonic reaction from Haldol. The patient continued to refuse fluids and was transferred to [other facility] to monitor input and output and dehydration. The patient had IV and Foley catheter. She was placed in four-point restraints due to her kicking the staff and not keeping her clothes on. On 3/26/89, the patient continued to refuse fluids or food. On 3/27/89, she was up and responding to verbal questioning. The patient cleaned herself up. While in the bathroom, the patient pulled out the IV and Foley. The patient began drinking fluids and her mother brought food from home. She began to eat the food brought from home well. The patient was transferred back to Receiving C. The patient became oriented and began to remember what had been happening in the last week. From 3/28/89 to 3/30/89, the patient continued to be cooperative, discussed stressors, and discussed mental illness. Arrangements were made to transfer the patient to [private hospital]. On 3/31/89, the patient was transferred to [private hospital] for continued hospitalization.

The next section is taken from the psychosocial history. The informants were Jenny's husband and her parents. Jenny was not interviewed herself "due to her extreme psychosis."

According to the informants, the patient found her natural childbirth experience frustrating due to her unrealistic expectations. The method that the patient chose conflicted with the standard hospital fetal monitoring techniques. This created numerous conflicts for the patient throughout the labor and delivery. Consequently, the patient left the hospital twelve hours after the birth, with the baby. The family indicated that the patient and her child were released appropriately, even though the physician recommended that they stay an additional one or two more days. The patient and the child were released under the care of the patient's mother, who provided the patient with rest and helped in caring for the newborn.

This is the patient's first psychiatric hospitalization. The onset was sudden, with a direct connection to the recent birth of her daughter. According to the informants, throughout the delivery of the child, the patient was hostile and suspicious of physicians. The patient had opted for a particular type of natural childbirth, three weeks prior to the birth of the baby. She discussed this with her obstetrician, who did not prepare her for certain discrepancies between hospital policy and the method of natural childbirth. The informants report that, even after the birth, the patient sustained her hostile and angry feelings.

The informants report that the symptoms escalated when the patient and her husband moved to [new state] in February of 1989. The husband hurt his back and could not help with the move and/or childcare. Therefore, the patient was left to cope with a new living situation in a new city, care of a newborn infant, and her first experience in moving away from her family. The family reported that the patient made statements to the effect that she could do it all, and did not need to eat or sleep, and that she was a very strong person. Resultant to this situation, the patient began to distort and exaggerate her religious philosophies and books that she was reading, interpreting these as "special messages from God." The patient began to make statements that she had heard the voice of God and began exhibiting confused behaviors. She would stare at the sun, believing that she was getting certain communications from God.

She read a book about allergies, and based upon certain chapters of this book, she threw out all of the plastic in the home, including the baby's bassinet, cleaning supplies, and turned off the heat. Because the baby had no place of its own to sleep, the child then slept with the patient and her husband, significantly interrupting the patient's sleep pattern to the extent that she did not sleep for several days. Also, based upon her reading, she refused to eat or drink anything but spring water. She has lost 20 pounds in three weeks. The patient sang religious hymns repetitively and was found on a public street in her underwear, staring at the sun. At this time, three days prior to her admission, the husband returned to [home state] with the patient and his daughter in order to seek the support of the patient's parents and assistance in obtaining mental health services.

After going to the private hospital, Jenny was sent back to the state hospital for her "uncooperative attitude" regarding the administration of medications. The next excerpts are from the discharge summary

DEPRESSION

---

from her second stay at the state hospital. It is during these six days that she went to court to try to avoid having to take antipsychotic medications.

Reason for admission: This 21 year old, white female was admitted on a Medical Certificate. She was transferred from [private hospital] because of her uncooperative behavior with the treatment. She was refusing to have any lab work done or comply with any medication. Before she was at [private hospital] she was at [state hospital]. Although she did go for a hearing and agreed to treatment, she did not cooperate when she went to [private hospital]. She has been for treatment. She has been having delusions.

Clinical course: The patient stayed on the Fourth Level until 4/18/89. She remained very uncooperative and guarded and paranoid. She was very much suspicious. She was very negative and was not responding to any questions. She was observed to be singing in the hallways and humming. She did not understand the need for treatment. She was approached for the physical examination and for the psychiatric evaluation almost every day. She did not cooperate very much except for the last few days. She was much more cooperative and did give some information. She provided that she had been acting very manic and hyperactive in the past. She agreed that she was doing some bizarre things. She has been scared and afraid and paranoid. Through the counseling she was willing to go to the private hospital and get treatment.

The next section is from the psychosocial history. The informants for this report are Jenny's parents. There is a great deal of overlap with the history reported at the time of first discharge. However, some differences provide additional information about her illness.

The patient is described as tending to be enthusiastic, generally does well at most things she attempts but tends to be "hard on herself if she finds herself falling short of her own expectations." She's considered to be very bright and creative, theatrically inclined and artistic. She enjoys being involved but tends to be very strong willed "not shy about expressing her opinions."

Although the family sees her emotional problems as starting on the day of daughter's delivery, the patient's obstetrician indicated that he thought he noticed manic symptoms approximately three weeks previously. [Note: he did not note these symptoms in her medical records, however.] The patient had planned on natural childbirth at [hospital name], in the birthing room, but at the time of the delivery became very angry when her doctor broke her waters and insisted on exercising certain hospital procedures which she objected to. She also was angry with her parents and husband for not backing her up, at the time of the birth there were five family members in the birthing room. The parents indicate that the patient was somewhat obsessed with having natural childbirth and that some of her expectations were unrealistic. The mother feels that she was not psychotic at the time of the birth, but did become so following her move to [another state]. The patient became even more inclined to believe what she read in various books, particularly being obsessed with a book on allergy, to the point she ran up considerable phone bills telling people to read the book then went on a three day fast, while nursing her baby. She started perceiving her husband as being evil and unclean because he works with computers and was not sympathetic to her expectations. It appears that her husband expressed some regrets at the idea of "never having a Big Mac or chocolate chip cookies again." She allegedly would not let her husband in the house on their anniversary because "God told me not to let you in." In several phone calls to her mother she said, "Satan is causing it."

ANALYSIS

The author of the psychosocial report apparently recognized that Jenny's illness had multiple causes. The report specifically mentions fatigue that was aggravated by and related to her mania, problems with social support brought on by her move to another state, and high expectations for herself as a wife and mother (wanting to be the best at everything). Fasting may have resulted in a metabolic imbalance that, in combination with other factors, triggered the psychosis. The lack of social support in the new town may have also allowed her illness to progress as far as it did.

What is particularly interesting is the apparent lack of understanding about the role of Jenny's childbirth experience in her illness by both her family and the people treating her. They viewed her expectations as "unrealistic." According to Jenny, clinicians at the state hospital tended to focus on her childbirth experience in some cases to the exclusion of all the other underlying factors. They focused on it while dismissing her feelings about it, as if naming her expectations as "unrealistic" would make her sense of disappointment and anger disappear. These issues and her perceptions of these events were important to her, however. Ironically, had her feelings been validated and had she been allowed to express them, her feelings of anger and disappointment could have dissipated. As it was, they continued to exert an influence.

INFORMATION ON PAST SEXUAL ABUSE

In 2001, four days after the death of Jenny's older brother, she started to have memories of being sexually abused as a baby surface. These memories were accompanied by a variety of sensations and feelings. She was rehospitalized in the summer of 2001 for a weekend of care for suicidal and homicidal feelings toward her perpetrator. During this time, she also had memories of being raped while in the state mental hospital on the first night of her arrival. She remembers being orally and vaginally assaulted by four orderlies while in four-point restraints, then taken to a seclusion room where she was thrown naked onto a mat. She has no evidence for these experiences except her memories and the fact that she developed oral herpes simplex II a few months after being released from the hospital. These assaults in the state hospital could explain her additional paranoia and fear while she was being treated. It also helps to explain her desire for death as well as periods of blackout and amnesia during certain points of her hospitalization.

THE ROAD TO RECOVERY

Jenny's recovery from her postpartum illness was a lengthy process. After her first stay in the private mental hospital, she was transferred back to the state hospital for six days. During this time, she went to court to avoid taking antipsychotic medication. The account of her continuing recovery is taken from an interview conducted for the first edition of this book.

During the six days back in the state mental hospital, I was literally a prisoner until I went to court. I had no friends, except for the other patients. Everyone was pressuring me. I called TV stations and reporters. One reporter was very supportive and wrote an article on postpartum depression. . . . While I was there, I was crazy. I'd sing patriotic songs and talk about my rights. During that time I was totally confused. I demanded a jury trial, which was my right. But they treated it like a joke. I wasn't a zombie.

My sentence was ninety days, forced medications if necessary. When I heard that, my heart literally broke. I couldn't fight it anymore. Back at the hospital, my mom yelled at me for three hours. She said that I had to take the drugs and come home and take care of my baby. I finally couldn't fight anymore.

I went back to the private hospital and started on lithium and Stelazine. I started to self-destruct and overeat. They told me it would "fix" the chemical imbalance in my brain. I didn't know [Stelazine] was a tranquilizer. When I started on the drugs, I was confused, couldn't finish a thought, tired (I slept sixteen to twenty hours a day), and depressed. The drugs worked though. They stopped the mania and racing thoughts. I'm not against drugs, only the improper use of drugs. Once I complied, I could do what I wanted. I was totally cooperative and even warm to my doctor, doing everything he said.

After two weeks in the private hospital, Jenny was released and stayed for five weeks at her parents' home. She then went home to her husband.

A big part of my recovery was going home to [new state] and facing my demons. I was worried about having no friends, about isolation. It was important to face what I was frightened of and being forced to be a mom again.

To help herself recover, she took her medications faithfully. She also began to put on weight and gained fifty pounds during that time. She started having severe PMS after coming home from the hospital. One psychiatrist told her she'd be on lithium for the rest of her life. That news was devastating. She called Depression After Delivery (DAD) and got a referral for a new psychiatrist. She went on progesterone, which helped with her PMS, and stopped lithium, but she was still on Stelazine. She started on Prozac and became very depressed. She was hospitalized again and was suicidal. Another doctor took her off Stelazine, which helped, and doubled her dosage of Prozac.

She identified several activities as helping her to recover. She started a support group for postpartum depression, was a DAD phone volunteer, and became a Bradley childbirth educator. "That was really important. Being around these happy couples who accepted me as a normal person." She had one twenty-minute flashback about a year after her release from the hospital. "That was scary. I thought I had beaten it. I didn't go on lithium or back in the hospital. It helped not to emphasize it." A pivotal moment came when she read an article in Newsweek about Prozac. It was then that she decided to try to wean herself away from the medications.

During that time, I was having highs and lows; really manic. I started looking for alternatives. During this time, I was obsessed with getting pregnant again to show I could do it right. I prayed. I discovered homeopathic, which cleanses the body. I discovered Chinese herbs. I feel this was from the Lord. Otherwise, I'd be on antidepressants again. It really helped. Going off of the drugs was like detox. I cried for a whole week. I think all the suppressed emotions of the last year came out.

I went through all the stages of grief, especially grief itself. It was so healing to have this time. I gained an additional fifty pounds. I didn't understand. I couldn't figure out what was happening until I read a book on detox—this is part of it. I still had severe PMS. I became a hermit. I was still obsessed with becoming pregnant, and I was somewhat depressed. Spiritually, I was completely depressed—I didn't want to talk to God. But it was a healing time, a happy time. I started to feel again. I could sing, feel joy, enjoy [my baby], my husband.

In January, I began a weight loss program with Chinese herbs and lost thirty pounds. I've paid lots of attention to nutrition. I have a semivegetarian lifestyle. I eat organic foods and drink distilled water. I've had no drugs for over a year. I use homeopathics, do yoga, and exercise faithfully.

Jenny has identified six factors that helped her heal. These included time to heal, the support of her husband, adequate nutrition (including fruits, vegetables, and dietary supplements), grieving over her lost time with her daughter, prayer of friends and family, and having another baby (thus moving on with her life).

Overall, Jenny is philosophical about her experience and feels that good has come of it. She summarized her feelings this way.

I don't regret that this happened. I don't feel bitter. I feel grateful to have had this experience. I didn't a year ago, but I do now. I feel empowered. Now I can empathize with other women, and I have placed myself in a key position to help other women. I don't know if I would have done this if I hadn't had this experience. I'd rather have had this experience than a normal easy birth. It uncluttered my life. It was the ultimate growth experience. I don't feel like I'm twenty-three, I feel like I'm fifty. I also feel that it was necessary. God allows things to happen to allow us to grow. Mental illness was not part of my plan, but it empowered me like nothing else could have to do what I needed to do.

2003 UPDATE

Jenny is now thirty-five. In the past twelve years, she has given birth to four additional children. Recognizing postpartum as a vulnerable time, she and her husband have taken extra precautions to ensure that she gets her rest and is not unduly stressed after childbirth. She has not experienced a relapse of her psychosis and has found alternatives to allopathic care.

Final Thoughts

As you can see, there is much you can do to help mothers suffering from postpartum depression. In surveying the whole of working with new mothers, I have a few final suggestions to help you on your way.

LISTEN TO MOTHERS

Whenever we know a lot about a subject, there is a natural tendency to want to share what we know with others. When dealing with depressed mothers, there is a time when it is appropriate to share what you know. But first, you should listen. Just letting a mother tell her story can be therapeutic in and of itself. It will also allow you time to figure out what the mother's real concerns might be. Sometimes mothers know and can articulate what is bothering them. They just need someone to hear them and validate what they are saying. Other mothers may not fully understand why they feel so bad. They just need to tell someone their story. I always know that I need to listen more when I start hearing "Yeah, but . . ." in response to a suggestion. If you listen, and the mother feels you have truly heard her, she will be more likely to follow your suggestions.

LET MOTHERS KNOW ABOUT FACTORS THAT MIGHT BE INFLUENCING THEIR EMOTIONAL STATES

After listening carefully, it is time to share what you know. Sometimes mothers really do not know why they feel bad. This can be true even years later. Dozens of times, I have been teaching a seminar and had participants come up and say that they never realized that a crying baby (or some other factor they identified with) could have caused their emotional distress. These women are generally health care professionals with grown children. Having someone simply name the factors involved can be validating to mothers and lets them know that they are not the only ones that have experienced what they are going through.

OFFER SPECIFIC SUGGESTIONS THAT CAN HELP

Once you have narrowed down the cause (or causes) of a mother's distress, offer her some strategies to alleviate the problem. For example, if she is in pain, teach her some ways to alleviate it (e.g., sitz baths, warm compresses, medications). If she is having breast pain, make an immediate referral to a lactation specialist to address the problem. If a mother is highly fatigued, brainstorm with her about how she can get more rest. Also be sure to rule out physical problems. If she has a baby with a difficult temperament, put her in contact with other mothers you know who have babies with this temperament. Self-help books can also be appropriate. Also be sure to rule out any physical cause of infant crying. Food sensitivities or gastroesophageal reflux are often culprits.

HELP MOTHERS MOBILIZE SUPPORT

Your role is pivotal in terms of helping mothers identify depression and referring them to the sources of help they need. But you cannot be a mother's long-term source of support. It is not practical and in the long run is not in the best interest of the mother. What you can do is help mothers find support among their own network and in their communities.

One of the most helpful things you can do is give mothers "permission" to get help and support. So often, mothers labor under the belief that they must tough things out themselves. Over the years, many mothers have related to me the apocryphal tale of the mother in the field who gives birth and gets right back to work. Yes, unfortunately, this does happen—especially in impoverished communities. But it is far from ideal. As I described in Chapter 7, it does not happen in many of the non-Western cultures with low rates of depression. In fact, I have found that just telling mothers about what happens in these cultures that support new mothers can be very liberating and encourages them to seek out support for themselves postpartum.

You might also have to refer mothers for other types of help. That means finding resources available in your community and even on-line. These types of resources can include support groups on various topics (breastfeeding, depression, difficult birth, premature babies, childbearing loss, mothering multiples, or single mothering). In rural communities, Web sites can be very helpful as specialized groups may not exist. Mothers may also need referrals for therapy and/or medications. Organizations such as Depression After Delivery and Postpartum Support International keep a list of professionals who specialize in the needs of postpartum women. State psychological or medical associations can also provide names of professionals in your community who can help depressed mothers. You may want to speak with these individuals before referring mothers, however. Also, be sure to find out what their payment policy is—especially for low-income mothers.

CONCLUSION

Intervention with new mothers can make a significant difference in their lives and the lives of their families. In closing, I would like to share the words of Salle Webber (1992), a postpartum doula who understands the pivotal role you can have in young families:

> Incredible as it seems, our culture, with its emphasis on education, has left young adults entirely unprepared to face the practical realities of parenting. And this may be the most important job they will ever hold. So, for those of us who are comfortable and happy in the work of parenting, we can serve the future of humanity through our humble sharing of our skills and our love for children and families. (p. 17)

I wish you great success in this important work.

References

Abou-Saleh, M.T., Ghubash, R., Karim, L., Krymski, M., & Bhai, I. (1998). Hormonal aspects of postpartum depression. *Psychoneuroendocrinology, 23,* 465-475.

Abraham, S., Taylor, A., & Conti, J. (2001). Postnatal depression, eating, exercise, and vomiting before and during pregnancy. *International Journal of Eating Disorders, 29,* 482-487.

Abramowitz, J., Moore, K., Carmin, C., Wiegartz, P.S., & Purdon, C. (2001). Acute onset of obsessive-compulsive disorder in males following childbirth. *Psychosomatics, 42,* 429-431.

Abramowitz, J.S., Schwartz, S.A., Moore, K.M., & Luenzmann, K.R. (2002). Obsessive-compulsive symptoms in pregnancy and the puerperium: A review of the literature. *Anxiety Disorders, 426,* 1-18.

Abramson, L.Y., Seligman, M.E.P., & Teasdale, J.D. (1978). Learned helplessness in humans: Critique and reformulation. *Journal of Abnormal Psychology, 87,* 49-74.

Affleck, G., Tennen, H., Rowe, J., Roscher, B., & Walker, L. (1989). Effects of formal support on mothers' adaptation to the hospital-to-home transition of high-risk infants: The benefits and costs of helping. *Child Development, 60,* 488-501.

Affonso, D.D., & Arizmendi, T.G. (1986). Disturbances in post-partum adaptation and depressive symptomatology. *Journal of Psychosomatic Obstetrics and Gynaecology, 5,* 15-32.

Affonso, D.D., De, A.K., Horowitz, J.A., & Mayberry, L.J. (2000). An international study exploring levels of postpartum depressive symptomatology. *Journal of Psychosomatic Research, 49,* 207-216.

Agency for Healthcare Research and Quality. (2002). *S-Adenosyl-L-Methionine for treatment of depression, osteoarthritis, and liver disease* (Evidence Report/ Technology Assessment No. 64). Rockville, MD: U.S. Department of Health and Human Services.

Ahokas, A., Aito, M., & Rimon, R. (2000). Positive treatment effect of estradiol in postpartum psychosis: A pilot study. *Journal of Clinical Psychiatry, 61,* 166-169.

Ahokas, A., Kaukoranta, J., Wahlbeck, K., & Aito, M. (2001). Estrogen deficiency in severe postpartum depression: Successful treatment with sublingual physiologic 17β estradiol: A preliminary study. *Journal of Clinical Psychiatry, 62,* 332-336.

Albertsson-Karlgren, U., Graff, M., & Nettelbladt, P. (2001). Mental disease postpartum and parent-infant interaction: Evaluation of videotaped sessions. *Child Abuse Review, 10,* 5-17.

Allgower, A., Wardle, J., & Steptoe, A. (2001). Depressive symptoms, social support, and personal health behaviors in young men and women. *Health Psychology, 20,* 223-227.

American Psychiatric Association. (2000) *Diagnostic and statistical manual of mental disorders* (4th ed., text rev.). Washington, DC: American Psychiatric Association.

Amir, L.H., Dennerstein, L., Garland, S.M., Fisher, J., & Farish, S.J. (1996). Psychological aspects of nipple pain in lactating women. *Journal of Psychosomatic Obstetrics and Gynecology, 17,* 53-58.

Anderson, G.C. (1991). Current knowledge about skin-to-skin (kangaroo) care for preterm infants. *Journal of Perinatology, 11,* 216-226.

Anderson, I.M., & Tomenson, B.M. (1995). Treatment discontinuation with selective serotonin reuptake inhibitors compared with tricyclic antidepressants: A meta-analysis. *British Medical Journal, 310,* 1433-1438.

Andreozzi, L., Flanagan, P., Seifer, R., Brunner, S., & Lester, B. (2002). Attachment classifications among 18-month-old children of adolescent mothers. *Archives of Pediatric and Adolescent Medicine, 156,* 20-26.

Anisfeld, E., Casper, V., Nozyce, M., & Cunningham, N. (1990). Does infant carrying promote attachment? An experimental study of the effects of increased physical contact on the development of attachment. *Child Development, 61,* 1617-1627.

Antonuccio, D. (1995). Psychotherapy for depression: No stronger medicine. *American Psychologist, 50,* 450-452.

Antonuccio, D., Danton, W.G., & DeNelsky, G.Y. (1995). Psychotherapy versus medication for depression: Challenging the conventional wisdom with data. *Professional Psychology: Research and Practice, 26,* 574-585.

Appleby, L., Mortensen, P.B., & Faragher, E.B. (1998). Suicide and other causes of mortality after postpartum psychiatric admission. *British Journal of Psychiatry, 173,* 209-211.

Appleby, L., Warner, R., Whitton, A., & Faragher, B. (1997). A controlled study of fluoxetine and cognitive-behavioral counseling in the treatment of postnatal depression. *British Medical Journal, 314,* 932-936.

Armstrong, K.L., Fraser, J.A., Dadds, M.R., & Morris, J. (1999). A randomized controlled trial of nurse home visiting to vulnerable families with newborns. *Journal of Paediatrics and Child Health, 35,* 237-244.

Ashman, S.B., Dawson, G., Panagiotides, H., Yamada, E., & Wilkins, C.W. (2002). Stress hormone levels of children of depressed mothers. *Development and Psychopathology, 14,* 333-349.

Astbury, J., Brown, S., Lumley, J., & Small, R. (1994). Birth events, birth experiences, and social differences in postnatal depression. *Australian Journal of Public Health, 18,* 176-184.

Avissar, S., Nechamkin, Y., Roitman, G., & Schreiber, G. (1997). Reduced G protein functions and immunoreactive levels in mononuclear leukocytes of patients with depression. *American Journal of Psychiatry, 154,* 211-217.

Ayers, S., & Pickering, A.D. (2001). Do women get posttraumatic stress disorder as a result of childbirth? A prospective study of incidence. *Birth, 28,* 111-118.

Babyak, M., Blumenthal, J.A., Herman, S., Khatri, P., Doraiswamy, M., Moore, K., Craighead, W.E., Baldewicz, T.T., & Krishnan, K.R. (2000). Exercise treatment for major depression: Maintenance of therapeutic benefit at 10 months. *Psychosomatic Medicine, 62,* 633-638.

Balch, P.A. (2002). *Prescription for herbal healing.* New York: Avery.

Barnett, B., & Parker, G. (1985). Professional and non-professional intervention for highly anxious primiparous mothers. *British Journal of Psychiatry, 146,* 287-293.

Baxter, L.R., Schwartz, J.M., Bergman, K.S., & Szuba, M.P. (1992). Caudate glucose metabolic rate changes with both drug and behavioral therapy for obsessive-compulsive disorders. *Archives of General Psychiatry, 49,* 681-689.

Beck, C.T. (1992). The lived experience of postpartum depression: A phenomenological study. *Nursing Research, 41,* 166-170.

Beck, C.T. (1993). Teetering on the edge: A substantive theory of postpartum depression. *Nursing Research, 42,* 42-48.

Beck, C.T. (1995). The effects of postpartum depression on maternal-infant interaction: A meta-analysis. *Nursing Research, 44,* 298-304.

Beck, C.T. (1996a). A meta-analysis of the relationship between postpartum depression and infant temperament. *Nursing Research, 45,* 225-230.

Beck, C.T. (1996b). Postpartum depressed mothers' experiences interacting with their children. *Nursing Research, 45,* 98-104.

Beck, C.T. (2001). Predictors of postpartum depression: An update. *Nursing Research, 50,* 275-285.

Beck, C.T. (2002). Postpartum depression: A metasynthesis. *Qualitative Health Research, 12,* 453-472.

Beck, C.T., & Gable, R.K. (2000). Postpartum Depression Screening Scale: Development and psychometric testing. *Nursing Research, 49,* 272-282.

Beck, C.T., & Gable, R.K. (2001a). Comparative analysis of the performance of the Postpartum Depression Screening Scale with two other depression instruments. *Nursing Research, 50,* 242-250.

Beck, C.T., & Gable, R.K. (2001b). Further validation of the Postpartum Depression Screening Scale. *Nursing Research, 50,* 155-164.

Beeghly, M., Weinberg, M.K., Olson, K.L., Kernan, H., Riley, J., & Tronick, E.Z. (2002). Stability and change in level of maternal depressive symptomatology during the first postpartum year. *Journal of Affective Disorders, 71,* 169-180.

Belizan, J.M., Althabe, F., Barros, F.C., & Alexander, S. (1999). Rates and implications of caesarean sections in Latin America: Ecological study. *British Medical Journal, 319,* 1397-1402.

Bendersky, M., & Lewis, M. (1986). The impact of birth order on mother-infant interactions in preterm and sick infants. *Journal of Developmental and Behavioral Pediatrics, 7,* 242-246.

Benedict, M., Paine, L., & Paine, L. (1994). *Long-term effects of child sexual abuse on functioning in pregnancy and pregnancy outcome.* Final report, National Center on Child Abuse and Neglect. Washington, DC: National Center on Child Abuse and Neglect.

Benedict, M.I., Paine, L.L., Paine, L.A., Brandt, D., & Stallings, R. (1999). The association of childhood sexual abuse with depressive symptoms during pregnancy, and selected pregnancy outcomes. *Child Abuse and Neglect, 23*, 659-670.

Bezchilibnzyk-Butler, K.Z., & Jeffries, J.J. (1999). *Clinical handbook of psychotropic drugs* (9th ed.). Seattle, WA: Hogrefe and Huber.

Bick, D.E., MacArthur, C., & Lancashire, R.J. (1998). What influences the uptake and early cessation of breastfeeding? *Midwifery, 14*, 242-247.

Black, M.M., Papas, M.A., Hussey, J.M., Dubowitz, H., Kotch, J.B., & Starr, R.H., Jr. (2002). Behavior problems among preschool children born to adolescent mothers: Effects of maternal depression and perceptions of partner relationships. *Journal of Clinical Child and Adolescent Psychology, 31*, 16-26.

Bladt, S., & Wagner, H. (1994). Inhibition of MAO by fractions and constituents of hypericum extract. *Journal of Geriatric Psychiatry and Neurology, 7* (Supplement), S57-S59.

Bloch, M., Schmidt, P.J., Danaceau, M., Murphy, J., Niemann, L., & Rubinow, D.R. (2000). Effects of gonadal steroids in women with a history of postpartum depression. *American Journal of Psychiatry, 157*, 924-930.

Blumberg, N.L. (1980). Effects of neonatal risk, maternal attitude, and cognitive style on early postpartum adjustment. *Journal of Abnormal Psychology, 89*, 139-150.

Blumenthal, M., Busse, W.R., Goldberg, A., Gruenwald, J., Hall, T., Riggins, C.W., et al. (Eds). (1998). *The Complete German Commission E Monographs: Therapeutic guide to herbal medicines.* Austin, TX: American Botanical Council.

Bond, M.J., Prager, M.A., Tiggemann, M., & Tao, B. (2001). Infant crying, maternal well-being and perceptions of caregiving. *Journal of Applied Health Behavior, 3*, 3-9.

Boukydis, C.F.Z., Lester, B.M., & Hoffman, J. (1987). Parenting and social support networks for parents of preterm and fullterm infants. In C.F.Z. Boukydis (Ed.), *Research on support for parents and infants in the postnatal period* (pp. 61-83). Norwood, NJ: Ablex.

Boyce, P., & Condon, J. (2001). Providing good clinical care means listening to women's concerns. *British Medical Journal, 322*, 928.

Boyce, P., Harris, M., Silove, D., Morgan, A., Wilhelm, K., & Hadzi-Pavlovic, D. (1998). Psychosocial factors associated with depression: A study of socially disadvantaged women with young children. *Journal of Nervous and Mental Disease, 186*, 3-11.

Bozoky, I., & Corwin, E.J. (2002). Fatigue as a predictor of postpartum depression. *Journal of Gynecologic, Obstetric, and Neonatal Nursing, 31*, 436-443.

Bratman, S., & Girman, A.M. (2003). *Handbook of herbs and supplements and their therapeutic uses.* St. Louis, MO: Mosby.

Bremner, J.D., Randall, P., Vermetten, E., Staib, L., Bronen, R.A., Mazure, C., Capelli, S., McCarthy, G., Innis, R.B., & Charney, D.S. (1997). Magnetic resonance imaging-based measurements of hippocampal volume in posttraumatic stress disorder related to childhood physical and sexual abuse: A preliminary report. *Biological Psychiatry, 41,* 23-32.

Brennan, P.A., Hammen, C., Anderson, M.J., Bor, W., Najman, J.M., & Williams, G.M. (2000). Chronicity, severity, and timing of maternal depressive symptoms: Relationships with child outcomes at age 5. *Developmental Psychology, 36,* 759-766.

Breslau, N., Chilcoat, H.D., Kessler, R.C., & Davis, G.C. (1999). Previous exposure to trauma and PTSD effects of subsequent trauma: Results from the Detroit Area Survey of Trauma. *American Journal of Psychiatry, 156,* 902-907.

Briere, J.N., & Elliot, D.M. (1994). Immediate and long-term impacts of child sexual abuse. *The Future of Children, 4,* 54-69.

Brown, M.-A., Goldstein-Shirley, J., Robinson, J., & Casey, S. (2001). The effects of multi-modal intervention trial on light, exercise, and vitamins on women's mood. *Women and Health, 34,* 93-112.

Brown, S., & Lumley, J. (2000). Physical health problems after childbirth and maternal depression at six to seven months postpartum. *British Journal of Obstetrics and Gynecology, 107,* 1194-1201.

Brown, S.L. (1996). Lowered serum cholesterol and low mood. *British Medical Journal, 313,* 637-638.

Brunner, J., Parhofer, K.G., Schwandt, P., & Bronisch, T. (2002). Cholesterol, essential fatty acids, and suicide. *Pharmacopsychiatry, 35,* 1-5.

Buist, A. (1998). Childhood abuse, postpartum depression and parenting difficulties: A literature review of associations. *Australian and New Zealand Journal of Psychiatry, 32,* 370-378.

Buist, A., & Janson, H. (2001). Childhood sexual abuse, parenting, and postpartum depression: A 3-year follow-up study. *Child Abuse and Neglect, 25,* 909-921.

Bullock, L.F.C., Libbus, M.K., & Sable, M.R. (2001). Battering and breastfeeding in a WIC population. *Canadian Journal of Nursing Research, 32,* 43-56.

Burns, D. (1999). *Feeling good: The new mood therapy.* New York: Avon.

Campbell, S.B., Cohn, J.F., Flanagan, C., Popper, S., & Meyers, T. (1992). Course and correlates of postpartum depression during the transition to parenthood. *Development and Psychopathology, 4,* 29-47.

Campeau, S., Day, H.E.W., Helmreich, D.L., Kollack-Walker, S., & Watston, S.J. (1998). Principles of psychoneuroendocrinology. *The Psychiatric Clinics of North America, 21,* 259-275.

Campos, J., Bartlett, K.C., Lamb, M.E., Goldsmith, H.H., & Stenberg, C. (1983). Socioemotional development. In P. Mussen (Ed.), *Handbook of child psychology* (4th ed., Vol. II, pp. 784-915). New York: Wiley.

Canivet, C., Jakobsson, I., & Hagander, B. (2002). Colicky infants according to maternal reports in telephone interviews and diaries: A large Scandinavian study. *Journal of Developmental and Behavioral Pediatrics, 23,* 1-8.

Capuzzi, C. (1989). Maternal attachment to handicapped infants and the relationship to social support. *Research in Nursing and Health, 12,* 161-167.

Cerutti, R., Sichel, M.P., & Perin, M. (1993). Psychological distress during puerperium: A novel therapeutic approach using S-adenosylmethionine. *Current Therapeutic Research, Clinical and Experimental, 53,* 707-716.

Chalmers, B.E., & Chalmers, B.M. (1986). Post-partum depression: A revised perspective. *Journal of Psychosomatic Obstetrics and Gynaecology, 5,* 93-105.

Chandra, P.S., Vankatasubramanian, G., & Thomas, T. (2002). Infanticidal ideas and infanticial behavior in Indian women with severe postpartum psychiatric disorders. *Journal of Nervous and Mental Disease, 190,* 457-461.

Charatan, F. (2002). Woman may face death penalty in postnatal depression case. *British Medical Journal, 324,* 634.

Chaudron, L.H., & Jefferson, J.W. (2001) Mood stabilizers during breastfeeding: A review. *Journal of Clinical Psychiatry, 61,* 79-90.

Chaudron, L.H., Klein, M.H., Remington, P., Palta, M., Allen, C., & Essex, M.J. (2001). Predictors, prodromes and incidence of postpartum depression. *Journal of Psychosomatic Obstetrics and Gynaecology, 22,* 103-112.

Cheasty, M., Clare, A.W., & Collins, C. (1998). Relation between sexual abuse in childhood and adult depression: Case-control study. *British Medical Journal, 316,* 198-201.

Chen, E., Bloomberg, G.R., Fisher, E.B., & Strunk, R.C. (2003). Predictors of repeat hospitalizations in children with asthma: The role of psychosocial and socioenvironmental factors. *Health Psychology, 22,* 12-18.

Cheruku, S.R., Montgomery-Downs, H.E., Farkas, S.L., Thoman, E.B., & Lammi-Keefe, C.J. (2002). Higher maternal plasma docosahexaenoic acid during pregnancy is associated with more mature neonatal sleep-state patterning. *American Journal of Clincial Nutrition, 76,* 608-613.

Chess, S., & Thomas, A. (1977). Temperamental individuality from childhood to adolescence. *Journal of Child Psychiatry, 16,* 218-226.

Chi, T.C., & Hinshaw, S.P. (2002). Mother-child relationships of children with ADHD: The role of maternal depressive symptoms and depression-related distortions. *Journal of Abnormal Child Psychology, 30,* 387-400.

Chung, T.K., Lau, T.K., Yip, A.S., Chiu, H.F., & Lee, D.T. (2001). Antepartum depressive symptomatology is associated with adverse obstetric and neonatal outcomes. *Psychosomatic Medicine, 63,* 830-834.

Cohen, L.S., Sichel, D.A., Dimmock, J.A., & Rosenbaum, J.F. (1994). Impact of pregnancy on panic disorder: A case series. *Journal of Clinical Psychiatry, 55,* 284-288.

Cohen, L.S., Viguera, A.C., Bouffard, S.M., Nonacs, R.M., Morabiot, C., Collins, M.H., & Ablon, J. S. (2001). Venlafaxine in the treatment of postpartum depression. *Journal of Clinical Psychiatry, 62,* 592-596.

Colegrave, S., Holcombe, C., & Salmon, P. (2001). Psychological characteristics of women presenting with breast pain. *Journal of Psychosomatic Research, 50,* 303-307.

Cooper, P.J., Landman, M., Tomlinson, M., Molteno, C., Swartz, L., & Murray, L. (2002). Impact of a mother-infant intervention in an indigent peri-urban South African context: Pilot study. *British Journal of Psychiatry, 180,* 76-81.

Cooper, P.J., & Murray, L. (1998). Postnatal depression. *British Medical Journal, 316,* 1884-1886.

Cooper, P.J., Tomlinson, M., Swartz, L., Woolgar, M., Murray, L., & Molteno, C. (1999). Postpartum depression and the mother-infant relationship in a South African peri-urban settlement. *British Journal of Psychiatry, 175,* 554-558.

Corral, M., Kuan, A., & Kostaras, D. (2000). Bright light therapy's effect on postpartum depression. *American Journal of Psychiatry, 157,* 303-304.

Corwin, E.J., Bozoky, I., Pugh, L.C., & Johnston, N. (2003). Interleukin-1 beta elevation during the postpartum period. *Annals of Behavioral Medicine, 25,* 41-47.

Coutu, M.F., Dupuis, G., & D'Antono, B. (2001). The impact of cholesterol lowering on patients' mood. *Journal of Behavioral Medicine, 24,* 517-536.

Cowan, C.P., & Cowan, P.A. (1987). A preventive intervention for couples becoming parents. In C.F.Z. Boukydis (Ed.), *Research on support for parents and infants in the postnatal period* (pp. 225-252). Norwood, NJ: Ablex.

Cox, J.L. (1988). Childbirth as a life event: Sociocultural aspects of postnatal depression. *Acta Psychiatrica Scandanavica Supplement, 344,* 75-83.

Cox, J.L., Connor, Y., & Kendell, R.E. (1982). Prospective study of the psychiatric disorders of childbirth. *British Journal of Psychiatry, 140,* 111-117.

Cox, J.L., Holden, J.M., & Sagovsky, R. (1987). Detection of postnatal depression: Development of the 10-item Edinburgh Postnatal Depression Scale. *British Journal of Psychiatry, 150,* 782-786.

Crnic, K., & Greenberg, M. (1987). Maternal stress, social support, and coping: Influences on the early mother-infant relationship. In C.F.Z. Boukydis (Ed.), *Research on support for parents and infants in the postnatal period* (pp. 25-41). Norwood, NJ: Ablex.

Crnic, K.A., Greenberg, M.T., & Slough, N.M. (1986). Early stress and social support influences on mothers' and high-risk infants' functioning in late infancy. *Infant Mental Health Journal, 7,* 19-33.

Crockenberg, S., & McCluskey, K. (1986). Change in maternal behavior during the baby's first year of life. *Child Development, 57,* 746-753.

Cryan, E., Keogh, F., Connolly, E., Cody, S., Quinlan, A., & Daly, I. (2001). Depression among postnatal women in an urban Irish community [Abstract]. *Irish Journal of Psychological Medicine, 18,* 5-10.

Cutrona, C.E. (1984). Social support and stress in the transition to parenthood. *Journal of Abnormal Psychology, 93,* 378-390.

Cutrona, C.E., & Troutman, B.R. (1986). Social support, infant temperament, and parenting self-efficacy: A mediational model of postpartum depression. *Child Development, 57,* 1507-1518.

Czarnocka, J., & Slade, P. (2000). Prevalence and predictors of posttraumatic stress symptoms following childbirth. *British Journal of Clinical Psychology, 39,* 35-51.

Da Costa, D., Dobkin, P.L., Dritsa, M., & Fitzcharles, M-A. (2001). The relationship between exercise participation and depressed mood in women with fibromyalgia. *Psychology, Health and Medicine, 6,* 301-311.

Da Costa, D., Larouche, J., Dritsa, M., & Brender, W. (2000). Psychosocial correlates of prepartum and postpartum depressed mood. *Journal of Affective Disorders, 59,* 31-40.

Dalton, K. (1985). Progesterone prophylaxis used successfully in postnatal depression. *Practitioner, 229,* 507-508.

Danaci, A.E., Dinc, G., Deveci, A., Sen, F.S., & Icelli, I. (2002). Postnatal depression in Turkey: Epidemiological and cultural aspects. *Social Psychiatry and Psychiatric Epidemiology, 37,* 125-129.

Dannenbring, D., Stevens, M.J., & House, A.E. (1997). Predictors of childbirth pain and maternal satisfaction. *Journal of Behavioral Medicine, 20,* 127-142.

Davidson, J., & Robertson, E. (1985). A follow-up study of post-partum illness, 1946-1978. *Acta Psychiatrica Scandanavica, 71,* 451-457.

DeRubeis, R.J., Gelfand, L.A., Tang, T.Z., & Simons, A.D. (1999). Medications versus cognitive behavior therapy for severely depressed outpatients: Meta-analysis of four randomized comparisons. *American Journal of Psychiatry, 156,* 1007-1013.

Des Rivieres-Pigeon, C., Seguin, L., Brodeur, J.-M., Perreault, M., Boyer, G., Colin, C., & Goulet, L. (2000). The Edinburgh Postnatal Depression Scale: Validity for Quebec women of low socioeconomic status. *Canadian Journal of Community Mental Health, 19,* 201-214.

Des Rivieres-Pigeon, C., Seguin, L., Goulet, L., & Descarries, F. (2001). Unraveling the complexities of the relationship between employment status and postpartum depressive symptomatology. *Women and Health, 34,* 61-79.

Devilly, G.J., & Spence, S.H. (1999). The relative efficacy and treatment distress of EMDR and cognitive behavioral trauma treatment protocol in the amelioration of posttraumatic stress disorder. *Journal of Anxiety Disorders, 13,* 131-158.

Diaz, A., Simatov, E., & Rickert, V.I. (2000). The independent and combined effects of physical and sexual abuse on health: Results of a national survey. *Journal of Pediatric and Adolescent Gynecology, 13,* 89.

DiLozenzo, T.M., Bargman, E.P., Stucky-Ropp, R., Brassington, G.S., Frensch, P.A., & LaFontaine, T. (1999). Long-term effects of aerobic exercise on psychological outcomes. *Preventive Medicine, 28,* 75-85.

Dodd, S., Stocky, A., Buist, A., Burrows, G.D., Maguire, K.I., & Norman, T.R. (2000). Sertraline in paired blood plasma and breast-milk samples from nursing mothers. *Human Psychopharmacology: Clinical and Experimental, 15,* 261-264.

Dombrowski, M.A., Anderson, G.C., Santori, C., & Burkhammer, M. (2001). Kangaroo (skin-to-skin) care with a postpartum woman who felt depressed. *MCN: American Journal of Maternal Child Nursing, 26,* 214-216.

Donovan, W.L., & Leavitt, L.A. (1989). Maternal self-efficacy and infant attachment: Integrating physiology, perceptions, and behavior. *Child Development, 60,* 460-472.

Donovan, W.L., Leavitt, L.A., & Walsh, R.O. (1990). Maternal self-efficacy: Illusory control and its effect on susceptibility to learned helplessness. *Child Development, 61,* 1638-1647.

Dubois, B. (2003 March-April). Overcoming the past. *New Beginnings,* 50-51.

Dubowitz, H., Black, M.M., Kerr, M.A., Hussey, J.M., Morrel, T.M., Everson, M.D., & Starr, R.H. (2001). Type and timing of mothers' victimization: Effects on mothers and children. *Pediatrics, 107,* 728-735.

Dudley, M., Roy, K., Kelk, N., & Bernard, D. (2001). Psychological correlates of depression in fathers and mothers in the first postnatal year. *Journal of Reproductive and Infant Psychology, 19,* 187-202.

Dunham, C. (1992). *Mamatoto: A celebration of birth.* New York: Viking Penguin.

Durik, A.M., Hyde, J.S., & Clark, R. (2000). Sequelae of cesarean and vaginal deliveries: Psychosocial outcomes for mothers and infants. *Developmental Psychology, 36,* 251-260.

Durrett, M.E., Otaki, M., & Richards, P. (1984). Attachment and the mother's perception of support from the father. *International Journal of Behavioral Development, 7,* 167-176.

Eberhard-Gran, M., Eskild, A., Tambs, K., Schei, B., & Opjordsmoen, S. (2001). The Edinburgh Postnatal Depression Scale: Validation in a Norwegian community sample [Abstract]. *Nordic Journal of Psychiatry, 55,* 113-117.

Edhborg, M., Lundh, W., Seimyr, L., & Widstroem, A.-M. (2001). The long-term impact of postnatal depressed mood on mother-child interaction: A preliminary study. *Journal of Reproductive and Infant Psychology, 19,* 61-71.

Eisenberg, A., Murkoff, H.E., & Hathaway, S.E. (1989). *What to expect the first year.* New York: Workman.

Elliot, S.A., & Leverton, T.J. (2000). Is the EPDS a magic wand? 2. "Myths" and the evidence base. *Journal of Reproductive and Infant Psychology, 18,* 297-307.

Elliot, S.A., Leverton, T.J., Sanjack, M., Turner, H., Cowmeadow, P., Hopkins, J., & Bushnell, D. (2000). Promoting mental health after childbirth: A controlled trial of primary prevention of postnatal depression. *British Journal of Clinical Psychology, 39,* 223-241.

Epel, E., Lapidus, R., McEwen, B., & Brownell, K. (2001). Stress may add bite to appetite in women: A laboratory study of stress-induced cortisol and eating behavior. *Psychoneuroendocrinology, 26,* 37-49.

Epperson, N., Czarkowski, K.A., Ward-O'Brien, D., Weiss, E., Gueorguieva, R., Jatlow, P., & Anderson, G.M. (2001). Maternal sertraline treatment and serotonin transport in breastfeeding mother-infant pairs. *American Journal of Psychiatry, 158,* 1631-1637.

Ernst, E. (2002). The risk-benefit profile of commonly used herbal therapies: Ginkgo, St. John's wort, ginseng, echinacea, saw palmetto, and kava. *Annals of Internal Medicine, 136,* 42-53.

Evans, J., Heron, J., Francomb, H., Oke, S., & Golding, J. (2001). Cohort study of depressed mood during pregnancy and after childbirth. *British Medical Journal, 323,* 257-260.

Feldman, R., Eidelman, A.I., Sirota, L., & Weller, A. (2002). Comparison of skin-to-skin (kangaroo) and traditional care: Parenting outcomes and preterm infant development. *Pediatrics, 110,* 16-26.

Felitti, V.J. (1991). Long-term medical consequences of incest, rape, and molestation. *Southern Medical Journal, 84,* 328-331.

Fergerson, S.S., Jamieson, D.J., & Lindsay, M. (2002). Diagnosing postpartum depression: Can we do better? *American Journal of Obstetrics and Gynecology, 186,* 899-902.

Fergusson, D.M., & Horwood, L.J. (1998). Exposure to interparental violence in childhood and psychosocial adjustment in young adulthood. *Child Abuse and Neglect, 22,* 339-357.

Field, T. (1992). Infants of depressed mothers. *Development and Psychopathology, 4,* 49-66.

Field, T. (1995). Infants of depressed mothers. *Infant Behavior and Development, 18,* 1-13.

Field, T. (1997). The treatment of depressed mothers and their infants. In L. Murray & P.J. Cooper (Eds.), *Postpartum depression and child development* (pp. 221-236). New York: Guilford.

Field, T., Diego, M., Hernandez-Reif, M., Schanberg, S., & Kuhn, C. (2002). Relative right versus left frontal EEG in neonates. *Developmental Psychobiology, 41,* 147-155.

Field, T., Fox, N.A., Pickens, J., & Nawrocki, T. (1995). Relative right frontal EEG activation in 3- to 6-month-old infants of "depressed" mothers. *Developmental Psychology, 31,* 358-363.

Figley, C.R. (1986). Traumatic stress: The role of the family and social support system. In C.R. Figley (Ed.), *Trauma and its wake:* Vol. 2: *Traumatic stress theory, research and intervention* (pp. 39-54). New York: Brunner/Mazel.

Fisher, J., Astbury, J., & Smith, A. (1997). Adverse psychological impact of operative obstetric interventions: A prospective longitudinal study. *Australian and New Zealand Journal of Psychiatry, 31,* 728-738.

Fisher, J.R., Feekery, C.J., Amir, L.H., & Sneddon, M. (2002). Health and social circumstances of women admitted to a private mother-baby unit. A descriptive cohort study. *Australian Family Physician, 31,* 966-970, 973.

Fisher, J.R.W., Feekery, C.J., & Rowe-Murray, H.J. (2002). Nature, severity and correlates of psychological distress in women admitted to a private mother-baby unit. *Journal of Paediatrics and Child Health, 38,* 140-145.

Fischer-Fay, F.A., Goldberg, S., Simmons, R., & Levison, H. (1988). Chronic illness and infant-mother attachment: Cystic fibrosis. *Journal of Developmental and Behavioral Pediatrics, 9,* 266-270.

Foa, E.B., & Cahill, S.P. (2002). Specialized treatment for PTSD: Matching survivors the appropriate modality. In R. Yehuda (Ed.), *Treating trauma survivors with PTSD* (pp. 43-62). Washington, DC: American Psychiatric Press.

Foss, G.F. (2001). Maternal sensitivity, posttraumatic stress, and acculturation in Vietnamese and Hmong mothers. *MCN, 26,* 257-263.

Franko, D.L., Blais, M.A., Becker, A.E., Delinsky, S.S., Greenwood, D.N., Flores, A.T., Ekelblad, E.R., Eddy, K.T., & Herzog, D.B. (2001). Pregnancy complications and neonatal outcomes in women with eating disorders. *American Journal of Psychiatry, 158,* 1461-1466.

Freeman, M.P. (2000). Omega-3 fatty acids in psychiatry: A review. *Annual Clinics in Psychiatry, 12,* 159-165.

Freeman, M.P., Smith, K.W., Freeman, S.A., McElroy, S.L., Kmetz, G.F., Wright, R., & Keck, P.E., Jr. (2002). The impact of reproductive events on the course of bipolar disorder in women. *Journal of Clinical Psychiatry, 63,* 284-287.

Friedman, M.J. (2001). *Posttraumatic stress disorder: The latest assessment and treatment strategies.* Kansas City, MO: Compact Clinicals.

Friedrich, W.N., & Sims, L.A. (2003, July). *Sexual abuse victims as mothers: Relationship to coping resources, perceptions of child, discipline practices, and behavior problems.* Paper presented at the 8th International Family Violence Research Conference, Portsmouth, New Hampshire.

Frodi, A., Bridges, L., & Shonk, S. (1989). Maternal correlates of infant temperament ratings and of infant-mother attachment: A longitudinal study. *Infant Mental Health Journal, 10,* 273-289.

Fuggle, P., Glover, L., Khan, F., & Haydon, K. (2002). Screening for postnatal depression in Bengali women: Preliminary observations from using a translated version of the Edinburgh Postnatal Depression Scale (EPDS). *Journal of Reproductive and Infant Psychology, 20,* 71-82.

Furman, L., Minich, N., & Hack, M. (2002). Correlates of lactation in mothers of very low birth weight infants. *Pediatrics, 109,* e57.

Galea, S., Vlahov, D., Resnick, H., Ahern, J., Susser, E., Gold, J., Bucuvalas, M., & Kilpatrick, D. (2003). Trends of probable post-traumatic stress disorder in New York City after the September 11 terrorist attacks. *American Journal of Epidemiology, 158*(6), 514-524.

Galler, J.R., Harrison, R.H., Biggs, M.A., Ramsey, F., & Forde, V. (1999). Maternal moods predict breastfeeding in Barbados. *Journal of Developmental and Behavioral Pediatrics, 20,* 80-87.

Galler, J.R., Harrison, R.H., Ramsey, F., Forde, V., & Butler, S.C. (2000). Maternal depressive symptoms affect infant cognitive development in Barbados. *Journal of Child Psychology and Psychiatry, 41,* 747-757.

Gamble, J.A., Creedy, D.K., Webster, J., & Moyle, W. (2002). A review of the literature on debriefing or non-directive counseling to prevent postpartum emotional distress. *Midwifery, 8*(1), 72-79.

Gaudin, J.M., Polansky, N.A., Kilpatrick, A.C., & Shilton, P. (1993). Loneliness, depression, stress, and social supports in neglectful families. *American Journal of Orthopsychiatry, 63,* 597-605.

Gaynes, B.N., Burns, B.J., Tweed, D.L., & Erickson, P. (2002). Depression and health-related quality of life. *Journal of Nervous and Mental Disease, 190*, 799-806.

Genevie, L., & Margolies, E. (1987). *The motherhood report: How women feel about being mothers.* New York: Macmillan.

Gjerdingen, D.K., & Chaloner, K.M. (1994). The relationship of women's postpartum mental health to employment, childbirth, and social support. *Journal of Family Practice, 38*, 465-472.

Glaser, R., Kiecolt-Glaser, J.K., Marucha, P.T., MacCallum, R.C., Laskowski, B.F., & Malarkey, W.B. (1999). Stress-related changes in proinflammatory cytokine production in wounds. *Archives of General Psychiatry, 56*, 450-456.

Gotlib, I.H., Whiffen, V.E., Wallace, P.M., & Mount, J.H. (1991). Prospective investigation of postpartum depression: Factors involved in onset and recovery. *Journal of Abnormal Psychology, 100*, 122-132.

Gracia, E., & Musitu, G. (2003). Social isolation from communities and child maltreatment: A cross-cultural comparison. *Child Abuse and Neglect, 27*, 153-168.

Grajeda, R., & Perez-Escamilla, R. (2002). Stress during labor and delivery is associated with delayed onset of lactation among urban Guatemalan women. *Journal of Nutrition, 132*, 3055-3060.

Grazioli, R., & Terry, D.J. (2000). The role of cognitive vulnerability and stress in the prediction of postpartum depressive symptomatology. *British Journal of Clinical Psychology, 39*, 329-347.

Grimstad, H., & Schei, B. (1999). Pregnancy and delivery for women with a history of child sexual abuse. *Child Abuse and Neglect, 23*, 81-90.

Guedeney, N., Fermanian, J., Guelfi, J.D., & Kumar, R.C. (2000). The Edinburgh Postnatal Depression Scale (EPDS) and the detection of major depressive disorders in early postpartum: Some concerns about false negatives. *Journal of Affective Disorders, 61*, 107-112.

Haapasalo, J., & Petaja, S. (1999). Mothers who killed or attempted to kill their child: Life circumstances, childhood abuse, and types of killing. *Violence and Victims, 14*, 219-239.

Hale, T. (2004). *Medications and mothers' milk* (10th ed.). Amarillo, TX: Pharmasoft.

Hammen, C., & Brennan, P. (2002). Interpersonal dysfunction in depressed women: Impairments independent of depressive symptoms. *Journal of Affective Disorders, 72*, 145-156.

Hannah, M.E., Hannah, W.J., Hodnett, E.D., Chalmers, B., Kung, R., Willan, A., Amankwah, K., Cheng, M., Helewa, M., Hewson, S., et al. (2002). Outcomes at 3 months after planned cesarean vs. planned vaginal delivery for breech presentation at term: The international randomized term breech trial. *Journal of the American Medical Association, 287*, 1822-1831.

Harkness, R., & Bratman, S. (2003). *Handbook of drug-herb and drug-supplement interactions.* St. Louis, MO: Mosby.

Harris, B., Fung, H., Johns, S., Kologlu, M., Bhatti, R., McGregor, A.M., Richards, C.J., & Hall, R. (1989). Transient post-partum thyroid dysfunction and postnatal depression. *Journal of Affective Disorders, 17,* 243-249.

Harris, B., Lovett, L., Newcombe, R.G., Read, G.F., Walker, R., & Riad-Fahmy, D. (1994). Maternity blues and major endocrine changes: Cardiff puerperal mood and hormone study II. *British Medical Journal, 308,* 949-953.

Hassmen, P., Koivula, N., & Uutela, A. (2000). Physical exercise and psychological well-being: A population study in Finland. *Preventive Medicine, 30,* 17-25.

Hay, D.F., & Kumar, R. (1995). Interpreting the effects of mothers' postnatal depression on children's intelligence: A critique and re-analysis. *Child Psychiatry and Human Development, 25,* 165-181.

Hay, D.F., Pawlby, S., Sharp, D., Asten, P., Mills, A., & Kumar, R. (2001). Intellectual problems shown by 11-year-old children whose mothers had postnatal depression. *Journal of Child Psychology and Psychiatry and Allied Disciplines, 42,* 871-889.

Hayes, B.A., Muller, R., & Bradley, B.S. (2001). Perinatal depression: A randomized controlled trial of an antenatal education intervention for primiparas. *Birth, 28,* 28-35.

Hayslip, C.C., Fein, H.G., O'Donnell, V.M., Friedman, D.S., Klein, T.A., & Smallridge, R.C. (1988). The value of serum antimicrosomal antibody testing in screening for symptomatic postpartum thyroid dysfunction. *American Journal of Obstetrics and Gynecology, 159,* 203-209.

Hearn, G., Iliff, A., Jones, I., Kirby, A., Ormiston, P., Parr, P., Rout, J., & Wardman, L. (1998). Postnatal depression in the community. *British Journal of General Practice, 48,* 1064-1066.

Heikkinen, T., Ekblad, U., Kero, P., Ekblad, S., & Laine, K. (2002). Citalopram in pregnancy and lactation. *Clinical Pharmacology and Therapeutics, 72,* 184-191.

Hendrick, V., Stowe, Z.N., Altshuler, L.L., Mintz, J., Hwang, S., Hostetter, A., Suri, R., Leight, K., & Fukuchi, A. (2001). Fluoxetine and norfluoxetine concentrations in nursing infants and breast milk. *Biological Psychiatry, 50,* 775-782.

Henry, O.A., Sheedy, M.T., & Beischer, N.A. (1989). When is a maternal death a maternal death? A review of maternal deaths at the Mercy Maternity Hospital, Melbourne. *Medical Journal of Australia, 151,* 628-631.

Hibbeln, J.R. (2002). Seafood consumption, the DHA content of mothers' milk and prevalence rates of postpartum depression: A cross-national, ecological analysis. *Journal of Affective Disorders, 69,* 15-29.

Hibbeln, J.R., Linnoila, M., Umhau, J.C., Rawlings, R., George, D.T., & Salem, N. (1998). Essential fatty acids predict metabolites of serotonin and dopamine in cerebrospinal fluid among healthy control subjects, and early- and late-onset alcoholics. *Biological Psychiatry, 44,* 235-242.

Hiscock, H., & Wake, M. (2002). Randomised controlled trial of behavioural infant sleep intervention to improve infant sleep and maternal mood. *British Medical Journal, 324,* 1062-1065.

Hobfoll, S.E., Ritter, C., Lavin, J., Hulsizer, M.R., & Cameron, R.P. (1995). Depression prevalence and incidence among inner-city pregnant and postpartum women. *Journal of Consulting and Clinical Psychology, 63*, 445-453.

Hoffman, Y., & Drotar, D. (1991). The impact of postpartum depressed mood on mother-infant interaction: Like mother like baby? *Infant Mental Health Journal, 12*, 65-80.

Hogberg, U., Innala, E., & Sandstrom, A. (1994). Maternal mortality in Sweden, 1980-1988. *Obstetrics and Gynecology, 84*, 240-244.

Holland, D. (2000). An observation of the effect of sertraline on breast milk supply. *Australian and New Zealand Journal of Psychiatry, 34*, 1032.

Horowitz, J.A., Bell, M., Trybulski, J.A., Munro, B.H., Moser, D., Hartz, S.A., McCordic, L., & Sokol, E.S. (2001). Promoting responsiveness between mothers with depressive symptoms and their infants. *Journal of Nursing Scholarship, 33*, 323-329.

House of Lords' Select Committee on Science and Technology. (2000). *Complementary and alternative medicine.* Available online at <http://www.parliament. the-stationery-office.co.uk/pa/ld199900/ldselect/ldsctech/123/12301.htm>.

Hughes, P., Turton, P., & Evans, C.D.H. (1999). Stillbirth as risk factor for depression and anxiety in the subsequent pregnancy: Cohort study. *British Medical Journal, 318*, 1721-1724.

Hulme, P.A. (2000). Symptomatology and health care utilization of women primary care patients who experienced childhood sexual abuse. *Child Abuse and Neglect, 24*, 1471-1484.

Hyde, J.S., Klein, M.H., Essex, M.J., & Clark, R. (1995). Maternity leave and women's mental health. *Psychology of Women Quarterly, 19*, 257-285.

Hypericum Depression Trial Study Group. (2002). Effect of *Hypericum perforatum* (St. John's wort) in major depressive disorder. *Journal of the American Medical Association, 287*, 1807-1814.

Ifabumuyi, O.I., & Akindele, M.O. (1985). Post-partum mental illness in northern Nigeria. *Acta Psychiatrica Scandinavica, 72*, 63-68.

Institute for Clinical Systems Improvement. (2004). *Health care guidelines: Major depression in specialty care in adults.* Available online at <www.icsi.org>.

Janssen, H.J., Cuisinier, M.C., Hoogduin, K.A., & de Graauw, K.P. (1996). Controlled prospective study on the mental health of women following pregnancy loss. *American Journal of Psychiatry, 153*, 226-230.

Jarvis, P.A., Myers, B.J., & Creasey, G.L. (1989). The effects of infants' illness on mothers' interactions with prematures at 4 and 8 months. *Infant Behavior and Development, 12*, 25-35.

Johnstone, S.J., Boyce, P.M., Hickey, A.R., Morris-Yates, A.D., & Harris, M.G. (2001). Obstetric risk factors for postnatal depression in urban and rural community samples. *Australian and New Zealand Journal of Psychiatry, 35*, 69-74.

Jones, I., & Craddock, N. (2001). Familiality of the puerperal trigger in bipolar disorder: Results of a family study. *American Journal of Psychiatry, 158*, 913-917.

Kalfus, M., & Shaffer, G. (1990, September 22). Newport woman jumps to her death at hotel. *The Orange County Register*, p. B1.

Kemeny, M.E., Weiner, H., Taylor, S.E., & Schneider, S. (1994). Repeated bereavement, depressed mood, and immune parameters in HIV seropostive and seronegative gay men. *Health Psychology, 13*, 14-24.

Kendall-Tackett, K.A. (2005). *The hidden feelings of motherhood: Coping with stress, depression, and burnout.* Amarillo, TX: Pharmasoft.

Kendell, R.E., Mackenzie, W.E., West, C., McGuire, R.J., & Cox, J.L. (1984). Day-to-day mood changes after childbirth: Further data. *British Journal of Psychiatry, 145*, 620-625.

Kendell, R.E., McGuire, R.J., Connor, J., & Cox, J.L. (1981). Mood changes in the first three weeks after childbirth. *Journal of Affective Disorders, 3*, 317-326.

Kimberling, R., Ouimette, P.C., Cronkite, R.C., & Moos, R. (2001). Depression and outpatient medical utilization: A naturalistic 10-year follow-up. *Annals of Behavioral Medicine, 21*, 317-321.

King, M., Davidson, O., Taylor, F., Haines, A., Sharp, D., & Turner, R. (2002). Effectiveness of teaching general practitioners skills in brief cognitive behavior therapy to treat patients with depression: Randomized controlled trial. *British Medical Journal, 324*, 947-950.

Kitzinger, S. (1990). *The crying baby.* London: Penguin.

Klier, C.M., Muzik, M., Rosenblum, K.L., & Lenz, G. (2001). Interpersonal psychotherapy adapted for the group setting in the treatment of postpartum depression. *Journal of Psychotherapy Practice and Research, 10*, 124-131.

Klier, C.M., Schafer, M.R., Schmid-Siegel, B., Lenz, G., & Mannel, M. (2002). St. John's wort *(Hypericum perforatum)*—Is it safe during breastfeeding? *Pharmacopsychiatry, 35*, 29-30.

Kuhn, M.A., & Winston, D. (2000). *Herbal therapy and supplements: A scientific and traditional approach.* Philadelphia, PA: Lippincott.

Lagana, L., Chen, X.-H., Koopman, C., Classen, C., Kimerling, R., & Spiegel, D. (2002). Depressive symptomatology in relation to emotional control and chronic pain in persons who are HIV positive. *Rehabilitation Psychology, 47*, 402-414.

Lane, A.M., Crone-Grant, D., & Lane, H. (2002). Mood changes following exercise. *Perceptual and Motor Skills, 94*, 732-734.

Lange, J.T., Lange, C.L., & Cabaltica, R.B.G. (2000). Primary care treatment of posttraumatic stress disorder. *American Family Physician, 62*, 1035-1040, 1046.

Lappin, J. (2001). Time points for assessing perinatal mood must be optimized. *British Medical Journal, 323*, 1367a.

Larsen, J.P., & Tandberg, E. (2001). Sleep disorders in patients with Parkinson's disease: Epidemiology and management. *CNS Drugs, 15*, 267-275.

Lavender, T., & Walkinshaw, S.A. (1998). Can midwives reduce postpartum psychological morbidity? A randomized trial. *Birth, 25*, 215-219.

Lawrence, R.A., & Lawrence, R.M. (1999). *Breastfeeding: A guide for the medical profession.* St. Louis, MO: Mosby.

Lecrubier, Y., Clerc, G., Didi, R., & Kieser, M. (2002). Efficacy of St. John's wort extract WS 5570 in major depression: A double-blind, placebo-controlled trial. *American Journal of Psychiatry, 159,* 1361-1366.

Lee, D.T., Yip, A.S., Chiu, H.F., & Chung, T.K. (2000). Screening for postnatal depression using a double-test strategy. *Psychosomatic Medicine, 62*(2), 258-263.

Lee, R.E., Goldberg, J.H., Sallis, J.F., Hickmann, S.A., Castro, C.M., & Chen, A.H. (2001). A prospective analysis of the relationship between walking and mood in sedentary ethnic minority women. *Women and Health, 32,* 1-15.

Leibenluft, E. (2000). Women and bipolar disorder: An update. *Bulletin of the Menninger Clinic, 64,* 5-17.

Leiferman, J. (2002). The effect of maternal depressive symptomatology on maternal behaviors associated with child health. *Health Education and Behavior, 29,* 596-607.

Leppaemaeki, S.J., Partonen, T.T., Hurme, J., Haukka, J.K., & Loennqvist, J.K. (2002). Randomized trial of the efficacy of bright-light exposure and aerobic exercise on depressive symptoms and serum lipids. *Journal of Clinical Psychiatry, 63,* 316-321.

Leserman, J., Petitto, J.M., Perkins, D.O., Folds, J.D., Golden, R.N., & Evans, D.L. (1997). Severe stress, depressive symptoms, and changes in lymphocyte subsets in human immunodeficiency virus-infected men: A 2-year follow-up study. *Archives of General Psychiatry, 54,* 279-285.

Lesperance, F., & Frasure-Smith, N. (2000). Depression in patients with cardiac disease: A practical review. *Journal of Psychosomatic Research, 48,* 379-391.

Leverton, T.J., & Elliot, S.A. (2000). Is the EPDS a magic wand? 1. A comparison of the Edinburgh Postnatal Depression Scale and health visitor report as predictors of diagnosis on the Present State Examination. *Journal of Reproductive and Infant Psychology, 18,* 279-296.

Levitt, M.J., Weber, R.A., & Clark, M.C. (1986). Social network relationships as sources of maternal support and well-being. *Developmental Psychology, 22,* 310-316.

Levy, V. (1987). The maternity blues in post-partum and post-operative women. *British Journal of Psychiatry, 151,* 368-372.

Lieb, R., Isensee, B., Hofler, M., Pfister, H., & Wittchen, H.-U. (2002). Parental major depression and the risk of depression and other mental disorders in offspring. *Archives of General Psychiatry, 59,* 365-374.

Linde, K., Ramirez, G., Mulrow, C.D., Pauls, A., Weidenhammer, W., & Melchart, D. (1996). St. John's wort for depression: An overview and meta-analysis of randomized clinical trials. *British Medical Journal, 313,* 253-258.

Lipman, T. (2002). The limitations of randomized controlled trials for socially constructed interventions. *British Medical Journal,* <bmj.bmjjournals.com/eletters/324/7345/1062>. Rapid responses for Hiscock and Wake, 324 (7345) 1062.

Lobel, M., DeVincent, C.J., Kaminer, A., & Meyer, B.A. (2000). The impact of prenatal maternal stress and optimistic disposition on birth outcomes in medically high-risk women. *Health Psychology, 19,* 544-553.

LoCicero, A.K., Weiss, D.M., & Issokson, D. (1997). Postpartum depression: Proposal for prevention through an integrated care and support network. *Applied and Preventive Psychology, 6,* 169-178.

Logsdon, M.C., & Usui, W. (2001). Psychosocial predictors of postpartum depression in diverse groups of women. *Western Journal of Nursing Research, 23,* 563-574.

Lucas, A., Pizarro, E., Granada, M.L., Salinas, I., & Santmarti, A. (2001). Postpartum thyroid dysfunction and postpartum depression: Are they two linked disorders? *Clinical Endocrinology, 55,* 809-814.

Luce, G.G. (1966). *Current research on sleep and dreams* (Public Health Service Publication No. 1389). Washington, DC: Public Health Service.

Luckas, M., Buckett, W., Aird, I., & Kingsland, C. (1997). Serum cholesterol concentration and postpartum depression. *British Medical Journal, 314,* 143.

Ludington-Hoe, S.M., with Golant, S.K. (1993). *Kangaroo care: The best you can do to help your preterm infant.* New York: Bantam.

Lumley, J., & Austin, M.-P. (2001). What interventions may reduce postpartum depression. *Current Opinion in Obstetrics and Gynecology, 13,* 605-611.

Lundy, B.L., Jones, N.A., Field, T., & Nearing, G. (1999). Prenatal depression effects on neonates. *Infant Behavior and Development, 22,* 119-129.

Luoma, I., Tamminen, T., Kaukonen, P., Laippala, P., Puura, K., Salelin, R., & Almqvist, F. (2001). Longitudinal study of maternal depressive symptoms and child well-being. *Journal of the American Academy of Child and Adolescent Psychiatry, 40,* 1367-1374.

Lutenbacher, M. (2002). Relationships between psychosocial factors and abusive parenting attitudes in low-income single mothers. *Nursing Research, 51,* 158-167.

Lutz, W.J., & Hock, E. (2002). Parental emotions following the birth of the first child: Gender differences in depressive symptoms. *American Journal of Orthopsychiatry, 72,* 415-421.

Lyons-Ruth, K., Connell, D.B., Grunebaum, H.U., & Botein, S. (1990). Infants at social risk: Maternal depression and family support services as mediators of infant development and security of attachment. *Child Development, 61,* 85-98.

MacArthur, C., Winter, H.R., Bick, D.E., Knowles, H., Lilford, R., Henderson, C., Lancashire, R.J., Braunholtz, D.A., & Gee, H. (2002). Effects of redesigned community postnatal care on women's health 4 months after birth: A cluster randomized controlled trial. *Lancet, 359,* 378-385.

MacLennan, A., Wilson, D., & Taylor, A. (1996). The self-reported prevalence of postnatal depression. *Australian and New Zealand Journal of Obstetric and Gynecology, 36,* 313.

Maes, M., Libbrecht, I., Lin, A.-H., Goossens, F., Ombelet, W., Stevens, K., Bosmans, E., Altamura, C., Cox, J., deJongh, R., & Scharpe, S. (2000). Effects of pregnancy and delivery on serum prolyl endopeptidase (PEP) activity: Alterations in serum PEP are related to increased anxiety in the early puerperium and to postpartum depression. *Journal of Affective Disorders, 57,* 125-137.

Maes, M., Lin, A.-H., Ombelet, W., Stevens, K., Kenis, G., deJongh, R., Cox, J., & Bosmans, E. (2000). Immune activation in the early puerperium is related to postpartum anxiety and depression symptoms. *Psychoneuroendocrinology, 25,* 121-137.

Maes, M., & Smith, R.S. (1998). Fatty acids, cytokines, and major depression. *Biological Psychiatry, 43,* 313-314.

Maina, G., Albert, U., Bogetto, F., Vaschetto, P., & Ravizza, L. (1999). Recent life events and obsessive-compulsive disorder (OCD): The role of pregnancy/delivery. *Psychiatry Research, 13,* 49-58.

Maloni, J.A., Kane, J.H., Suen, L.J., & Wang, K.K. (2002). Dysphoria among high-risk pregnant hospitalized women on bed rest: A longitudinal study. *Nursing Research, 51,* 92-99.

Manber, R., Allen, J.J., & Morris, M.M. (2002). Alternative treatments for depression: Empirical support and relevance to women. *Journal of Clinical Psychiatry, 63,* 628-640.

Mandl, K.D., Tronick, E.Z., Brennan, T.A., Alpert, H.R., & Home, C.J. (1999). Infant health care use and maternal depression. *Archives of Pediatric and Adolescent Medicine, 153,* 808-813.

Manning, J.S. (2002). *The brain-body connection and the relationship between depression and pain.* Available online at <www.medscape.com/viewprogram/2166_pnt>.

Mantle, F. (2002). The role of alternative medicine in treating postnatal depression. *Complementary Therapies in Nursing and Midwifery, 8,* 197-203.

Marcus, D.A. (2000). Treatment of nonmalignant chronic pain. *American Family Physician, 61,* 1331-1338.

Marcus, R., Panhuysen, G., Tuiten, A., & Koppeschaar, H. (2000). Effects of food on cortisol and mood in vulnerable subjects under controllable and uncontrollable stress. *Physiological Behavior, 70,* 333-342.

Markus, C.R., Panhuysen, G., Tuiten, A., Koppeschaar, H., Fekkes, D., & Peters, M.L. (1998). Does carbohydrate-rich, protein-poor feed prevent a deterioration of mood and cognitive performance of stress-prone subjects when subjected to a stressful event? *Appetite, 31,* 49-65.

Marshall, P. (1993). Allergy and depression: A neurochemical threshold model of the relation between the illnesses. *Psychological Bulletin, 113,* 23-43.

Martinez, R., Johnston-Robledo, I., Ulsh, H.M., & Chrisler, J.C. (2000). Singing "the baby blues": A content analysis of popular press articles about postpartum affective disturbances. *Women and Health, 31,* 37-56.

Mather, A.S., Rodriguez, C., Guthrie, M.F., McHarg, A.M., Reid, I.C., & Mc-Murdo, M.E.T. (2002). Effects of exercise on depressive symptoms in older adults with poorly responsive depressive disorder: Randomized controlled trial. *British Journal of Psychiatry, 180,* 411-415.

Mathews, C., & Baker, C. (2002). Responding to a baby's cries. *British Medical Journal,* <bmj.bmjjournals.com/eletters/324/7345/1062>. Rapid responses for Hiscock and Wake, 324 (7345) 1062.

Matthey, S., Barnett, B., Kavanagh, D.J., & Howie, P. (2001). Validation of the Edinburgh Postnatal Depression Scale for men, and comparison of item endorsement with their partners. *Journal of Affective Disorders, 64*(2-3), 175-184.

Matthey, S., Barnett, B., Ungerer, J., & Waters, B. (2000). Paternal and maternal depressed mood during the transition to parenthood. *Journal of Affective Disorders, 60,* 75-85.

McGrath, E., Keita, G.P., Strickland, B.R., & Russo, N.F. (1990). *Women and depression: Risk factors and treatment issues.* Washington, DC: American Psychological Association.

McKee, M.D., Cunningham, M., Jankowski, K.R., & Zayas, L. (2001). Health-related functional status in pregnancy: Relationship to depression and social support in a multi-ethnic population. *Obstetrics and Gynecology, 97,* 988-993.

McKim, M.K., Cramer, K.M., Stuart, B., & O'Connor, D.L. (1999). Infant care decisions and attachment security: The Canadian Transition to Child Care study. *Canadian Journal of Behavioural Science, 31,* 92-106.

McLennan, J.D., & Kotelchuck, M. (2000). Parental prevention practices for young children in the context of maternal depression. *Pediatrics, 105,* 1090-1095.

McLennan, J.D., Kotelchuck, M., & Cho, H. (2001). Prevalence, persistence, and correlates of depressive symptoms in a national sample of mothers of toddlers. *Journal of the American Academy of Child and Adolescent Psychiatry, 40,* 1316-1323.

McLennan, J.D., & Offord, D.R. (2002). Should postpartum depression be targeted to improve child mental health? *Journal of the American Academy of Child and Adolescent Psychiatry, 41,* 28-35.

Meyer, C.L., & Oberman, M. (2001). *Mothers who kill their children: Understanding the acts of moms from Susan Smith to the "Prom Mom."* New York: NYU Press.

Mezzacappa, E.S., & Katkin, E.S. (2002). Breastfeeding is associated with reduced perceived stress and negative mood in mothers. *Health Psychology, 21,* 187-193.

Mick, E., Biederman, J., Prince, J., Fischer, B.A., & Faraone, S.V. (2002). Impact of low birth weight on attention-deficit hyperactivity disorder. *Journal of Developmental and Behavioral Pediatrics, 23,* 16-22.

Miller, A.H. (1998). Neuroendocrine and immune system interactions in stress and depression. *Psychiatric Clinics of North America, 21,* 443-463.

Miller, L.J. (2002). Postpartum depression. *Journal of the American Medical Association, 287,* 762-765.

Mirowsky, J., & Ross, C.E. (2002). Depression, parenthood, and age at first birth. *Social Science and Medicine, 54*, 1281-1298.

Misri, S., Kim, J., Riggs, K.W., & Kostaras, X. (2000). Paroxetine levels in postpartum depressed women, breast milk, and infant serum. *Journal of Clinical Psychiatry, 61*, 828-832.

Misri, S., Kostaras, X., Fox, D., & Kostaras, D. (2000). The impact of partner support in the treatment of postpartum depression. *Canadian Journal of Psychiatry, 45*, 554-558.

Misri, S., Sinclair, D.A., & Kuan, A.J. (1997). Breastfeeding and postpartum depression: Is there a relationship? *Canadian Journal of Psychiatry, 42*, 1061-1065.

Moline, M.L., Kahn, D.A., Ross, R.W., Altshuler, L.L., & Cohen, L.S. (2001, March). Postpartum depression: A guide for patients and families. *Postgraduate Medicine Special Report*, 112-113.

Moore, G.A., Cohn, J.F., & Campbell, S.B. (2001). Infant affective responses to mother's still face at 6 months differentially predict externalizing and internalizing behaviors at 18 months. *Developmental Psychology, 37*, 706-714.

Morrell, C.J., Spiby, H., Stewart, P., Walters, S., & Morgan, A. (2000). Costs and effectiveness of community postnatal support workers: Randomised controlled trial. *British Medical Journal, 321*, 593-598.

Morris-Rush, J.K., & Bernstein, P.S. (2002). Postpartum depression. *Medscape Ob/Gyn and Women's Health*. <www.medscape.com/viewarticle/433013>.

Mu, P.-F., Wong, T.-T., Chang, K.-P., & Kwan, S.-Y. (2001). Predictors of maternal depression for families having a child with epilepsy. *Journal of Nursing Research, 9*, 116-126.

Murray, C.J.L., & Lopez, A.D. (1997). Global mortality, disability, and the contribution of risk factors: Global Burden of Disease Study. *Lancet, 349*, 1436-1442.

Murray, L., Stanley, C., Hooper, R., & King, F. (1996). The role of infant factors in postnatal depression and mother-infant interactions. *Developmental Medicine and Child Neurology, 38*, 109-119.

Murray, L., Woolgar, M., Cooper, P., & Hipwell, A. (2001). Cognitive *vulnerability* to depression in 5-year-old children of depressed mothers. *Journal of Child Psychology and Psychiatry, 42*, 891-899.

Mynors-Wallis, L.M., Gath, D.H., Day, A., & Baker, F. (2000). Randomized controlled trial of problem solving treatment, antidepressant medication, and combined treatment for major depression in primary care. *British Medical Journal, 320*, 26-30.

Mynors-Wallis, L.M., Gath, D.H., Lloyd-Thomas, A.R., & Tomlinson, D. (1995). Randomized controlled trial comparing problem solving treatment with amitriptyline and placebo for major depression in primary care. *British Medical Journal, 310*, 441-445.

Najman, J.M., Williams, G.M., Nikles, J., Spence, S., Bor, W., O'Callaghan, M., LeBrocque, R., & Andersen, M.J. (2000). Mothers' mental illness and child behavior problems: Cause-effect association or observation bias? *Journal of the American Academy of Child and Adolescent Psychiatry, 39,* 592-602.

Nelson, E.C., Heath, A.C., Madden, P.A.F., Cooper, L., Dinwiddie, S.H., Bucholz, K.K., Glowinski, A., McLaughlin, T., Dunne, M.P., Statham, D.J., et al. (2002). Association between self-reported childhood sexual abuse and adverse psychological outcomes: Results from a twin study. *Archives of General Psychiatry, 59,* 139-145.

Nicholas, L., Dawkins, K., & Golden, R.N. (1998). Psychoneuroendocrinology of depression: Prolactin. *Psychiatric Clinics of North America, 21,* 341-357.

Novosad, C., Freudigman, K., & Thoman, E.B. (1999). Sleep patterns in newborns and temperament at eight months: A preliminary study. *Journal of Developmental and Behavioral Pediatrics, 20,* 99-105.

Oakley, A. (1983). Social consequences of obstetric technology: The importance of measuring "soft" outcomes. *Birth, 10,* 99-108.

O'Connor, T.G., Thorpe, K., Dunn, J., & Golding, J. (1999). Parental divorce and adjustment in adulthood: Findings from a community sample. *Journal of Child Psychology and Psychiatry and Allied Disciplines, 40,* 777-789.

O'Hara, M.W. (1986). Social support, life events, and depression during pregnancy and the puerperium. *Archives of General Psychiatry, 43,* 569-573.

O'Hara, M.W. (1987). Post-partum "blues," depression, and psychosis: A review. Special issue: Maternal development during reproduction. *Journal of Psychosomatic Obstetrics and Gynaecology, 7,* 205-227.

O'Hara, M.W. (1994). Postpartum depression: Identification and measurement in a cross-cultural context. In J. Cox & J. Holden (Eds.), *Perinatal psychiatry: Use and misuse of the Edinburgh Postnatal Depression Scale* (pp. 145-168). London: Gaskell Press.

O'Hara, M.W. (1995). *Postpartum depression: Causes and consequences.* New York: Springer-Verlag.

O'Hara, M.W., Neunaber, D.J., & Zekoski, M. (1984). A prospective study of postpartum depression: Prevalence, course and predictive factors. *Journal of Abnormal Psychology, 93,* 158-171.

O'Hara, M.W., Rehm, L.P., & Campbell, S.B. (1983). Postpartum depression: A role for social network and life stress variables. *Journal of Nervous Disorders, 171,* 336-341.

O'Hara, M.W., Schlechte, J.A., Lewis, D.A., & Varner, M.W. (1991). Controlled prospective study of postpartum mood disorders: Psychological, environmental, and hormonal variables. *Journal of Abnormal Psychology, 100,* 63-73.

O'Hara, M.W., Stuart, S., Gorman, L.L., & Wenzel, A. (2000). Efficacy of interpersonal psychotherapy for postpartum depression. *Archives of General Psychiatry, 57,* 1039-1045.

O'Hara, M.W., & Swain, A.M. (1996). Rates and risk of postpartum depression: A meta-analysis. *International Review of Psychiatry, 8,* 37-54.

O'Rourke, D.A., Wurtman, J.J., Wurtman, R.J., Tsay, R., Gleason, R., Baer, L., & Jenike, M.A. (1994). Aberrant snacking patterns and eating disorders in patients with obsessive compulsive disorder. *Journal of Clinical Psychiatry, 55,* 445-447.

Ozalp, G., Sarioglu, R., Tuncel, G., Aslan, K.I., & Kadiogullari, N. (2003). Preoperative emotional states in patients with breast cancer and postoperative pain. *Acta Anaesthesiolica Scandinavica, 47,* 26-29.

Pajulo, M., Savonlahti, E., Sourander, A., Ahlqvist, S., Helenius, H., & Piha, J. (2001). An early report on the mother-baby interactive capacity of substance-abusing mothers. *Journal of Substance Abuse Treatment, 20,* 143-151.

Pajulo, M., Savonlahti, E., Sourander, A., Helenius, H., & Piha, J. (2001). Antenatal depression, substance dependency, and social support. *Journal of Affective Disorders, 65,* 9-17.

Parry, B.L., Curran, M.L., Stuenkel, C.A., Yokimozo, M., Tam, L., Powell, K.A., & Gillin, J.C. (2000). Can critically timed sleep deprivation be useful in pregnancy and postpartum depression? *Journal of Affective Disorders, 60,* 201-212.

Patel, V., Abas, M., Broadhead, J., Todd, C., & Reeler, A. (2001). Depression in developing countries: Lesson from Zimbabwe. *British Medical Journal, 322,* 482-484.

Patel, V., Rodrigues, M., & DeSouza, N. (2002). Gender, poverty, and postnatal depression: A study of mothers in Goa, India. *American Journal of Psychiatry, 159,* 43-47.

Pauli-Pott, U., Becker, K., Mertesacker, T., & Beckmann, D. (2000). Infants with "colic"—Mothers' perspectives on the crying problem. *Journal of Psychosomatic Research, 48,* 125-132.

Pauli-Pott, U., Darui, A., & Beckman, D. (1999). Infants with atopic dermatitis: Maternal hopelessness, child-rearing attitudes and perceived infant temperament. *Psychotherapy and Psychosomatics, 68,* 39-45.

Pedersen, C. (1999). Postpartum mood and anxiety disorders: A guide for the nonpsychiatric clinician with an aside on thyroid associations with postpartum mood. *Thyroid, 9,* 691-697.

Peet, M., & Horrobin, D.F. (2002). A dose-ranging study of the effects of ethyl-eicosapentaenoate in patients with ongoing depression despite apparently adequate treatment with standard drugs. *Archives of General Psychiatry, 59,* 913-919.

Peet, M., Murphy, B., Shay, J., & Horrobin, D. (1998). Depletion of omega-3 fatty acid levels in red blood cell membranes of depressive patients. *Biological Psychiatry, 43,* 315-319.

Perl, F.M. (2002). Infant sleep intervention or Nazi drill? *British Medical Journal,* <bmj.bmjjournals.com/eletters/324/7345/1062>. Rapid responses for Hiscock and Wake 324 (7345), 1062.

Peter, E.A., Janssen, P.A., Grange, C.S., & Douglas, M.J. (2001). Ibuprofen versus acetaminophen with codeine for the relief of perineal pain after childbirth: A randomized controlled trial. *Canadian Medical Association Journal, 165,* 1203-1209.

Philipp, M., Kohnen, R., & Hiller, K.-O. (1999). Hypericum extract versus imipramine or placebo in patients with moderate depression: Randomized multicenter study of treatment for eight weeks. *British Medical Journal, 319,* 1534-1539.

Piontek, C.M., Baab, S., Peindl, K.S., & Wisner, K.L. (2000). Serum valproate levels in 6 breastfeeding mother-infant pairs. *Journal of Clinical Psychiatry, 61,* 170-172.

Piontek, C.M., Wisner, K.L., Perel, J.M., & Peindl, K.S. (2001). Serum fluvoxamine levels in breastfed infants. *Journal of Clinical Psychiatry, 62,* 111-113.

Ploeckinger, B., Dantendorfer, K., Ulm, M., Baischer, W., Derfler, K., Musalek, M., & Dadak, L. (1996). Rapid decrease of serum cholesterol concentration and post-partum depression. *British Medical Journal, 313,* 664.

Pratt, L.A., Ford, D.E., Crum, R.M., Armenian, H.K., Gallo, J.J., & Eaton, W.W. (1996). Depression, psychotropic medication, and risk of myocardial infarction. Prospective data from the Baltimore ECA follow-up. *Circulation, 94,* 3123-3129.

Prentice, J.C., Lu, M.C., Lange, L., & Halfon, N. (2002). The association between reported childhood sexual abuse and breastfeeding initiation. *Journal of Human Lactation, 18,* 219-226.

Preston, J., & Johnson, J. (2004). *Clinical psychopharmacology made ridiculously simple, Edition 5.* Miami, FL: MedMaster.

Puri, B.K., Counsell, S.J., Hamilton, G., Richardson, A.J., & Horrobin, D.F. (2001). Eicosapentaenoic acid in treatment-resistant depression associated with symptom remission, structural brain changes and reduced neuronal phospholipids turnover. *International Journal of Clinical Practice, 55,* 560-563.

Quinn, T.J., & Carey, G.B. (1999). Does exercise intensity or diet influence lactic acid accumulation in breast milk? *Medicine and Science in Sports and Exercise, 31,* 105-110.

Rapkin, A.J., Mikacich, J.A., Moatakef-Imani, B., & Rasgon, N. (2002). The clinical nature and formal diagnosis of premenstrual, postpartum, and perimenopausal affective disorders. *Current Psychiatry Reports, 4,* 419-428.

Reading, R., & Reynolds, S. (2001). Debt, social disadvantage and maternal depression. *Social Science and Medicine, 53,* 441-453.

Regmi, S., Sligl, W., Carter, D., Grut, W., & Seear, M. (2002). A controlled study of postpartum depression among Nepalese women: Validation of the Edinburgh Postpartum Depression Scale in Kathmandu. *Tropical Medicine and International Health, 7,* 378-382.

Remick, R.A. (2002). Diagnosis and management of depression in primary care: A clinical update and review. *Canadian Medical Association Journal, 167,* 253-260.

Reynolds, J.L. (1997). Posttraumatic stress disorder after childbirth: The phenomenon of traumatic birth. *Canadian Medical Association Journal, 156,* 831-835.

Rhoades, N., & Hutchinson, S. (1994). Labor experiences of child sexual abuse survivors. *Birth, 21,* 213-220.

Righetti-Veltema, M., Conne-Perreard, E., Bousquet, A., & Manzano, J. (2002). Postpartum depression and mother-infant relationship at 3 months old. *Journal of Affective Disorders, 70,* 291-306.

Riley, D., & Eckenrode, J. (1986). Social ties: Subgroup differences in costs and benefits. *Journal of Personality and Social Psychology, 51,* 770-778.

Ritter, C., Hobfoll, S.E., Lavin, J., Cameron, R.P., & Hulsizer, M.R. (2000). Stress, psychosocial resources, and depressive symptomatology during pregnancy in low-income, inner-city women. *Health Psychology, 19,* 576-585.

Roberts, J., Sword, W.S., Gafni, A., Krueger, P., Sheehan, D., & Soon-Lee, K. (2001). Costs of postpartum care: Examining associations from the Ontario mother and infant survey. *Canadian Journal of Nursing Research, 33,* 19-34.

Rosenblum, K.L., McDonough, S., Muzik, M., Miller, A., & Sameroff, A. (2002). Maternal representations of the infant: Associations with infant response to the still face. *Child Development, 73,* 999-1015.

Rothman, B.K. (1982). *Giving birth: Alternatives in childbirth.* New York: Penguin.

Rowe-Murray, H.J., & Fisher, J.R.W. (2001). Operative intervention in delivery is associated with compromised early mother-infant interaction. *British Journal of Obstetrics and Gynaecology, 108,* 1068-1075.

Rowe-Murray, H.J., & Fisher, J.R.W. (2002). Baby friendly hospital practices: Cesarean section is a persistent barrier to early initiation of breastfeeding. *Birth, 29,* 124-131.

Saisto, T., Salmela-Aro, K., Nurmi, J.E., & Halmesmaki, E. (2001). Psychosocial predictors of disappointment with delivery and puerperal depression: A longitudinal study. *Acta Obstetrica et Gynecologica Scandinavica, 80,* 39-45.

Salmela-Aro, K., Nurmi, J.-E., Saisto, T., & Halmesmaki, E. (2001). Goal reconstruction and depressive symptoms during the transition to motherhood: Evidence from two cross-lagged longitudinal studies. *Journal of Personality and Social Psychology, 81,* 1144-1159.

Salovey, P., Rothman, A.J., Detweiler, J.B., & Steward, W.T. (2000). Emotional states and physical health. *American Psychologist, 55,* 110-121.

Sapolsky, R.M. (2000). Glucocorticoids and hippocampal atrophy in neuropsychiatric disorders. *Archives of General Psychiatry, 57,* 925-935.

Sayar, K., Arikan, M., & Yontem, T. (2002). Sleep quality in chronic pain patients. *Canadian Journal of Psychiatry, 47,* 844-848.

Sayegh, R., Schiff, I., Wurtman, J., Spiers, P., McDermott, J., & Wurtman, R. (1995). The effect of a carbohydrate-rich beverage on mood, appetite, and cognitive function in women with premenstrual syndrome. *Obstetrics and Gynecology, 86,* 520-528.

Schmidt, K., Olesen, O.V., & Jensen, P.N. (2000). Citalopram and breastfeeding: Serum concentration and side effects in the infant. *Biological Psychiatry, 47,* 164-165.

Schneider, M.S. (2001). *Pain: Perception and management.* Mountain View, CA: Cortext.

Schwartz, K., D'Arcy, H.J., Gillespie, B., Bobo, J., Longeway, M., & Foxman, B. (2002). Factors associated with weaning in the first 3 months postpartum. *Journal of Family Practice, 51,* 439-444.

Scott, D. (1987). Maternal and child health nurse: Role in post-partum depression. *Australian Journal of Advanced Nursing, 5,* 28-37.

Seng, J.S., Oakley, D.J., Sampselle, C.M., Killion, C., Graham-Bermann, S., & Liberzon, I. (2001). Posttraumatic stress disorder and pregnancy complications. *Obstetrics and Gynecology, 97,* 17-22.

Severus, W.E., Littman, A.B., & Stoll, A.L. (2001). Omega-3 fatty acids, homocysteine, and the increased risk of cardiovascular mortality in major depressive disorder. *Harvard Review of Psychiatry, 9,* 280-293.

Shields, N., Reid, M., & Cheyne, H. (1997). Impact of midwife-managed care in the postnatal period: An exploration of psychosocial outcomes. *Journal of Reproductive and Infant Psychology, 15,* 91-108.

Sichel, D.A., Cohen, L.S., Dimmock, J.A., & Rosenbaum, J.F. (1993). Postpartum obsessive compulsive disorder: A case series. *Journal of Clinical Psychiatry, 54,* 156-159.

Silvers, K.M., & Scott, K.M. (2002). Fish consumption and self-reported physical and mental health status. *Public Health Nutrition, 5,* 427-431.

Simkin, P. (1991). Just another day in a woman's life? Women's long-term perceptions of their first birth experience. Part I. *Birth, 18,* 203-210.

Simkin, P. (1992). Just another day in a woman's life? Part II: Nature and consistency of women's long-term memories of their first birth experiences. *Birth, 19,* 64-81.

Simon, G., Ormel, J., VonKorff, M., & Barlow, W. (1995). Health care costs associated with depressive and anxiety disorders in primary care. *American Journal of Psychiatry, 152,* 352-357.

Simon, G.E., VonKorff, M., Rutter, C., & Wagner, E. (2000). Randomised trial of monitoring, feedback, and management of care by telephone to improve treatment of depression in primary care. *British Medical Journal, 320,* 550-554.

Simopoulos, A.P. (2002). Omega-3 fatty acids in inflammation and autoimmune diseases. *Journal of the American College of Nutritionists, 21,* 495-505.

Singh, N.A., Clements, K.M., & Fiatarone Singh, M.A. (2001). The efficacy of exercise as a long-term antidepressant in elderly subjects: A randomized, controlled trial. *Journal of Gerontology, 56A,* M497-M504.

Skinner, E. (1991). My experience with PPP. *Heart Strings: The National Newsletter of Depression After Delivery, 2,* 1-2.

Small, R., Lumley, J., Donohue, L., Potter, A., & Waldenstrom, U. (2000). Randomised controlled trial of midwife led debriefing to reduce maternal depression after operative childbirth. *British Medical Journal, 321,* 1043-1047.

Smyke, A.T., Boris, N.W., & Alexander, G.M. (2002). Fear of spoiling in at-risk African American mothers. *Child Psychiatry and Human Development, 32,* 295-307.

Spinelli, M.G. (1998). Psychiatric disorders during pregnancy and postpartum. *Journal of the American Medical Women's Association, 53,* 165-170.

Stefos, G., Staner, L., Kerkhofs, M., Hubain, P., Mendlewicz, J., & Linkowski, P. (1998). Shortened REM latency as a psychobiological marker for psychotic depression? An age-, gender-, and polarity-controlled study. *Biological Psychiatry, 15,* 1314-1320.

Stein, A., Woolley, H., Murray, L., Cooper, P., Cooper, S., Noble, F., Affonso, N., & Fairburn, C.G. (2001). Influence of psychiatric disorder on the controlling behavior of mothers with 1-year-old infants: A study of women with maternal eating disorder, postnatal depression and a healthy comparison group. *British Journal of Psychiatry, 179,* 157-162.

Stern, G., & Kruckman, L. (1983). Multi-disciplinary perspectives on post-partum depression: An anthropological critique. *Social Science and Medicine, 17,* 1027-1041.

Stoll, A.L., Severus, W.E., Freeman, M.P., Rueter, S., Zboyan, H.A., Diamond, E., Cress, K.K., & Marangell, L.B. (1999). Omega-3 fatty acids in bipolar disorder: A preliminary double-blind, placebo-controlled trial. *Archives of General Psychiatry, 56,* 407-412.

Stuart, S., Couser, G., Schilder, K.I., & O'Hara, M.W. (1998). Postpartum anxiety and depression: Onset and comorbidity in a community sample. *Journal of Nervous and Mental Disease, 186,* 420-424.

Stuart, S., & O'Hara, M.W. (1995). Interpersonal psychotherapy for postpartum depression. *Journal of Psychotherapy Practice and Research, 4,* 18-29.

Taj, R., & Sikander, K.S. (2003). Effects of maternal depression on breastfeeding. *Journal of the Pakistani Medical Association, 53,* 8-11.

Thomas, A., & Chess, S. (1987). Commentary. In H.H. Goldsmith, A.H. Buss, R. Plomin, M.K. Rothbart, A. Thomas, S. Chess, R.R. Hinde, & R.B. McCall (Eds.), Roundtable: What is temperament? Four approaches. *Child Development, 58,* 505-529.

Thompson, J.F., Roberts, C.L., Currie, M., & Ellwood, D.A. (2002). Prevalence and persistence of health problems after childbirth: Associations with parity and method of birth. *Birth, 29,* 83-94.

Tolman, A.O. (2001). *Depression in adults: The latest assessment and treatment strategies.* Kansas City, MO: Compact Clinicals.

Toufexis, A. (1988, June 20). Why mothers kill their babies. *Time,* 81-83.

Troisi, A., Moles, A., Panepuccia, L., Lo Russo, D., Palla, G., & Scucchi, S. (2002). Serum cholesterol levels of mood symptoms in the postpartum period. *Psychiatry Research, 109,* 213-219.

Tronick, E.Z., & Weinberg, M.K. (1997). Depressed mothers and infants: Failure to form dyadic states of consciousness. In L. Murray & P. Cooper (Eds.), *Postpartum depression and child development* (pp. 54-81). New York: Guilford.

U.S. Census Bureau. (1998). *The official statistics.* Available online at <www.census.gov>.

van der Kolk, B.A. (2002). Assessment and treatment of complex PTSD. In R. Yehuda (Ed.), *Treating trauma survivors with PTSD* (pp. 127-156). Washington, DC: American Psychiatric Press.

van Gurp, G., Meterissian, G.B., Haiek, L.N., McCusker, J., & Bellavance, F. (2002). St. John's wort or sertraline? Randomized controlled trial in primary care. *Canadian Family Physician, 48,* 905-912.

VanderMeer, Y.G., Loendersloot, E.W., & VanLoenen, A.C. (1984). Effect of high-dose progesterone in post-partum depression. *Journal of Psychosomatic Obstetrics and Gynaecology, 3,* 67-68.

Veddovi, M., Kenny, D.T., Gibson, F., Bowen, J., & Starte, D. (2001). The relationship between depressive symptoms following premature birth, mothers' coping style, and knowledge of infant development. *Journal of Reproductive and Infant Psychology, 19,* 313-323.

Verdoux, H., Sutter, A.L., Glatigny-Dallay, E., & Minisini, A. (2002). Obstetrical complications and the development of postpartum depressive symptoms: A prospective survey of the MATQUID cohort. *Acta Psychiatrica Scandanavica, 106,* 212-219.

Wambach, K.A. (1998). Maternal fatigue in breastfeeding primiparae during the first nine weeks postpartum. *Journal of Human Lactation, 14,* 219-229.

Watson, E., & Evans, S.J. (1986). An example of cross-cultural measurement of psychological symptoms in postpartum mothers. *Social Science and Medicine, 23,* 869-874.

Watson, J.P., Elliot, S.A., Rugg, A.J., & Brough, D.I. (1984). Psychiatric disorder in pregnancy and the first postnatal year. *British Journal of Psychiatry, 144,* 453-462.

Webber, S. (1992). Supporting the postpartum family. *The Doula, 23,* 16-17.

Webster, J., Linnane, J.W.J., Dibley, L.M., Hinson, J.K., Starrenburg, S.E., & Roberts, J.A. (2000). Measuring social support in pregnancy: Can it be simple and meaningful? *Birth, 27,* 97-101.

Webster, J., Linnane, J.W.J., Dibley, L.M., & Pritchard, M. (2000). Improving antenatal recognition of women at risk for postnatal depression. *Australia and New Zealand Journal of Obstetrics and Gynaecology, 40,* 409-412.

Webster, J., Linnane, J., Dibley, L., Starrenburg, S., Roberts, J., & Hinson, J. (1997). The impact of screening for risk factors associated with postnatal depression at the first prenatal visit. *Journal of Quality Clinical Practice, 17,* 65-71.

Webster, J., Pritchard, M.A., Linnane, J.W., Roberts, J.A., Hinson, J.K., & Starrenburg, S.E. (2001). Postnatal depression: Use of health services and satisfaction with healthcare providers. *Journal of Quality Clinical Practice, 21,* 144-148.

Weetman, A.P. (1997). Fortnightly review. Hypothyroidism: Screening and subclinical disease. *British Medical Journal, 314,* 1175-1178.

Weinberg, M.K., & Tronick, E.Z. (1998). Emotional characteristics of infants associated with maternal depression and anxiety. *Pediatrics, 102*(Suppl.), 1298-1304.

Weinberg, M.K., Tronick, E.Z., Beeghly, M., Olson, K.L., Kernan, H., & Riley, J.M. (2001). Subsyndromal depressive symptoms and major depression in postpartum women. *American Journal of Orthopsychiatry, 71,* 87-97.

Weinraub, M., & Wolf, B. (1987). Stress, social supports and parent-child interactions: Similarities and differences in single-parent and two-parent families. In C.F.Z. Boukydis (Ed.), *Research on support for parents and infants in the postnatal period* (pp. 84-113). Norwood, NJ: Ablex.

Wertz, R.W., & Wertz, D.C. (1989). *Lying in: A history of childbirth in America* (Expanded ed.). New Haven, CT: Yale University Press.

Whiffen, V.E. (1990). Maternal depressed mood and perceptions of child temperament. *Journal of Genetic Psychology, 151,* 329-339.

Whiffen, V.E., & Gotlib, I.H. (1989). Infants of postpartum depressed mothers: Temperament and cognitive status. *Journal of Abnormal Psychology, 98,* 274-279.

Whiskey, E., Werneke, U., & Taylor, D. (2001). A systematic review and meta-analysis of *Hypericum perforatum* in depression: A comprehensive clinical review. *International Clinical Psychopharmacology, 16,* 239-252.

Williams, K.E., & Koran, L.M. (1997). Obsessive-compulsive disorder in pregnancy, the puerperium, and the premenstruum. *Journal of Clinical Psychiatry, 58,* 330-334.

Williamson, G.M., Walters, A.S., & Shaffer, D.R. (2002). Caregiver models of self and others, coping, and depression: Predictors of depression in children with chronic pain. *Health Psychology, 21,* 405-410.

Wilson, J.P., & Zigelbaum, S.D. (1986). Post-traumatic stress disorder and the disposition to criminal behavior. In C.R. Figley (Ed.), *Trauma and its wake: Traumatic stress theory, research, and intervention* (Vol. II, pp. 305-322). New York: Brunner/Mazel.

Wisner, K.L., Peindl, K.S., Gigliotti, T., & Hanusa, B.H. (1999). Obsessions and compulsions in women with postpartum depression. *Journal of Clinical Psychiatry, 60,* 176-180.

Wisner, K.L., Perel, J.M., & Findling, R.L. (1996). Antidepressant treatment during breastfeeding. *American Journal of Psychiatry, 153,* 1132-1137.

Wisner, K.L., Perel, J.M., Peindl, K.S., Hanusa, B.H., Findling, R.L., & Rapport, D. (2001). Prevention of recurrent postpartum depression: A randomized clinical trial. *Journal of Clinical Psychiatry, 62,* 82-86.

Wolf, A.W., De Andraca, I., & Lozoff, B. (2002). Maternal depression in three Latin American samples. *Social Psychiatry and Psychiatric Epidemiology, 37,* 169-176.

Wolke, D., Rizzo, P., & Woods, S. (2002). Persistent infant crying and hyperactivity problems in middle childhood. *Pediatrics, 109,* 1054-1060.

Worrall, G., Angel, J., Chaulk, P., Clarke, C., & Robbins, M. (1999). Effectiveness of an educational strategy to improve family physicians' detection and management of depression: A randomized controlled trial. *Canadian Medical Association Journal, 161,* 37-40.

Wurtman, J.J., Brzezinski, A., Wurtman, R.J., & Laferrere, B. (1989). Effect of nutrient intake on premenstrual depression. *American Journal of Obstetrics and Gynecology, 161,* 1228-1234.

Wurtman, J.J., & Suffes, S. (1997). *The serotonin solution to achieve permanent weight control.* New York: Columbine.

Wurtman, R.J., & Wurtman, J.J. (1995). Brain serotonin, carbohydrate-craving, obesity and depression. *Obesity Research, 3*(Suppl.), 477S-480S.

Wurtman, R.J., Wurtman, J.J., Regan, M.M., McDermott, J.M., Tsay, R.H., & Breu, J.J. (2003). Effects of normal meals rich in carbohydrates or proteins on plasma tryptophan and tyrosine ratios. *American Journal of Clinical Nutrition, 77,* 128-132.

Xu, Z., & Lu, B. (2001). Relationship between postpartum depression, life events, and social support [Abstract]. *Chinese Journal of Clinical Psychology, 9,* 130, 132.

Yamashita, H., Yoshida, K., Nakano, H., & Tashiro, N. (2000). Postnatal depression in Japanese women: Detecting the early onset of postnatal depression by closely monitoring the postpartum mood. *Journal of Affective Disorders, 58,* 145-154.

Yonkers, K.A., Ramin, S.M., Rush, A.J., Navarrete, C.A., Carmody, T., March, D., Heartwell, S.F., & Leveno, K.J. (2001). Onset and persistence of postpartum depression in an inner-city maternal health clinic system. *American Journal of Psychiatry, 158,* 1856-1863.

Zelkowitz, P., & Milet, T.H. (2001). The course of postpartum psychiatric disorders in women and their partners. *Journal of Nervous and Mental Disease, 189,* 575-582.

Index

Page numbers followed by the letter "b" indicate boxed material; those followed by the letter "t" indicate tables.

CHILD MALTREATMENT RISK ASSESSMENTS: AN EVALUATION GUIDE by Sue Righthand, Bruce Kerr, and Kerry Drach. (2003). "This book is essential reading for clinicians and forensic examiners who see cases involving issues related to child maltreatment. The authors have compiled an impressive critical survey of the relevant research on child maltreatment. Their material is well organized into sections on definitions, impact, risk assessment, and risk management. This book represents a giant step toward promoting evidence-based evaluations, treatment, and testimony." *Diane H. Schetky, MD, Professor of Psychiatry, University of Vermont College of Medicine*

SIMPLE AND COMPLEX POST-TRAUMATIC STRESS DISORDER: STRATEGIES FOR COMPREHENSIVE TREATMENT IN CLINICAL PRACTICE edited by Mary Beth Williams and John F. Sommer Jr. (2002). "A welcome addition to the literature on treating survivors of traumatic events, this volume possesses all the ingredients necessary for even the experienced clinician to master the management of patients with PTSD." *Terence M. Keane, PhD, Chief, Psychology Service, VA Boston Healthcare System; Professor and Vice Chair of Research in Psychiatry, Boston University School of Medicine*

FOR LOVE OF COUNTRY: CONFRONTING RAPE AND SEXUAL HARASSMENT IN THE U.S. MILITARY by T. S. Nelson. (2002). "Nelson brings an important message—that the absence of current media attention doesn't mean the problem has gone away; that only decisive action by military leadership at all levels can break the cycle of repeated traumatization; and that the failure to do so is, as Nelson puts it, a 'power failure'—a refusal to exert positive leadership at all levels to stop violent individuals from using the worst power imaginable." *Chris Lombardi, Correspondent, Women's E-News, New York City*

THE INSIDERS: A MAN'S RECOVERY FROM TRAUMATIC CHILDHOOD ABUSE by Robert Blackburn Knight. (2002). "An important book. . . . Fills a gap in the literature about healing from childhood sexual abuse by allowing us to hear, in undiluted terms, about one man's history and journey of recovery." *Amy Pine, MA, LMFT, psychotherapist and co-founder, Survivors Healing Center, Santa Cruz, California*

WE ARE NOT ALONE: A GUIDEBOOK FOR HELPING PROFESSIONALS AND PARENTS SUPPORTING ADOLESCENT VICTIMS OF SEXUAL ABUSE by Jade Christine Angelica. (2002). "Encourages victims and their families to participate in the system in an effort to heal from their victimization, seek justice, and hold offenders accountable for their crimes. An exceedingly vital training tool." *Janet Fine, MS, Director, Victim Witness Assistance Program and Children's Advocacy Center, Suffolk County District Attorney's Office, Boston*

WE ARE NOT ALONE: A TEENAGE GIRL'S PERSONAL ACCOUNT OF INCEST FROM DISCLOSURE THROUGH PROSECUTION AND TREATMENT by Jade Christine Angelica. (2002). "A valuable resource for teens who have been sexually abused and their parents. With compassion and eloquent prose, Angelica walks people through the criminal justice system—from disclosure to final outcome." *Kathleen Kendall-Tackett, PhD, Research Associate, Family Research Laboratory, University of New Hampshire, Durham*

WE ARE NOT ALONE: A TEENAGE BOY'S PERSONAL ACCOUNT OF CHILD SEXUAL ABUSE FROM DISCLOSURE THROUGH PROSECUTION AND TREATMENT by Jade Christine Angelica. (2002). "Inspires us to work harder to meet kids' needs, answer their questions, calm their fears, and protect them from their abusers and the system, which is often not designed to respond to them in a language they understand." *Kevin L. Ryle, JD, Assistant District Attorney, Middlesex, Massachusetts*

GROWING FREE: A MANUAL FOR SURVIVORS OF DOMESTIC VIOLENCE by Wendy Susan Deaton and Michael Hertica. (2001). "This is a necessary book for anyone who is scared and starting to think about what it would take to 'grow free.' . . . Very helpful for friends and relatives of a person in a domestic violence situation. I recommend it highly." *Colleen Friend, LCSW, Field Work Consultant, UCLA Department of Social Welfare, School of Public Policy & Social Research*

A THERAPIST'S GUIDE TO GROWING FREE: A MANUAL FOR SURVIVORS OF DOMESTIC VIOLENCE by Wendy Susan Deaton and Michael Hertica. (2001). "An excellent synopsis of the theories and research behind the manual." *Beatrice Crofts Yorker, RN, JD, Professor of Nursing, Georgia State University, Decatur*

PATTERNS OF CHILD ABUSE: HOW DYSFUNCTIONAL TRANSACTIONS ARE REPLICATED IN INDIVIDUALS, FAMILIES, AND THE CHILD WELFARE SYSTEM by Michael Karson. (2001). "No one interested in what may well be the major public health epidemic of our time in terms of its long-term consequences for our society can afford to pass up the opportunity to read this enlightening work." *Howard Wolowitz, PhD, Professor Emeritus, Psychology Department, University of Michigan, Ann Arbor*

IDENTIFYING CHILD MOLESTERS: PREVENTING CHILD SEXUAL ABUSE BY RECOGNIZING THE PATTERNS OF THE OFFENDERS by Carla van Dam. (2000). "The definitive work on the subject. . . . Provides parents and others with the tools to recognize when and how to intervene." *Roger W. Wolfe, MA, Co-Director, N. W. Treatment Associates, Seattle, Washington*

POLITICAL VIOLENCE AND THE PALESTINIAN FAMILY: IMPLICATIONS FOR MENTAL HEALTH AND WELL-BEING by Vivian Khamis. (2000). "A valuable book . . . a pioneering work that fills a glaring gap in the study of Palestinian society." *Elia Zureik, Professor of Sociology, Queens University, Kingston, Ontario, Canada*

STOPPING THE VIOLENCE: A GROUP MODEL TO CHANGE MEN'S ABUSIVE ATTITUDES AND BEHAVIORS by David J. Decker. (1999). "A concise and thorough manual to assist clinicians in learning the causes and dynamics of domestic violence." *Joanne Kittel, MSW, LICSW, Yachats, Oregon*

STOPPING THE VIOLENCE: A GROUP MODEL TO CHANGE MEN'S ABUSIVE ATTITUDES AND BEHAVIORS, THE CLIENT WORKBOOK by David J. Decker. (1999).

BREAKING THE SILENCE: GROUP THERAPY FOR CHILDHOOD SEXUAL ABUSE, A PRACTITIONER'S MANUAL by Judith A. Margolin. (1999). "This book is an extremely valuable and well-written resource for all therapists working with adult survivors of child sexual abuse." *Esther Deblinger, PhD, Associate Professor of Clinical Psychiatry, University of Medicine and Dentistry of New Jersey School of Osteopathic Medicine*

"I NEVER TOLD ANYONE THIS BEFORE": MANAGING THE INITIAL DISCLOSURE OF SEXUAL ABUSE RE-COLLECTIONS by Janice A. Gasker. (1999). "Discusses the elements needed to create a safe, therapeutic environment and offers the practitioner a number of useful strategies for responding appropriately to client disclosure." *Roberta G. Sands, PhD, Associate Professor, University of Pennsylvania School of Social Work*

FROM SURVIVING TO THRIVING: A THERAPIST'S GUIDE TO STAGE II RECOVERY FOR SURVIVORS OF CHILDHOOD ABUSE by Mary Bratton. (1999). "A must read for all, including survivors. Bratton takes a lifelong debilitating disorder and unravels its intricacies in concise, succinct, and understandable language." *Phillip A. Whitner, PhD, Sr. Staff Counselor, University Counseling Center, The University of Toledo, Ohio*

SIBLING ABUSE TRAUMA: ASSESSMENT AND INTERVENTION STRATEGIES FOR CHILDREN, FAMILIES, AND ADULTS by John V. Caffaro and Allison Conn-Caffaro. (1998). "One area that has almost consistently been ignored in the research and writing on child maltreatment is the area of sibling abuse. This book is a welcome and required addition to the developing literature on abuse." *Judith L. Alpert, PhD, Professor of Applied Psychology, New York University*

BEARING WITNESS: VIOLENCE AND COLLECTIVE RESPONSIBILITY by Sandra L. Bloom and Michael Reichert. (1998). "A totally convincing argument. . . . Demands careful study by all elected representatives, the clergy, the mental health and medical professions, representatives of the media, and all those unwittingly involved in this repressive perpetuation and catastrophic global problem." *Harold I. Eist, MD, Past President, American Psychiatric Association*

TREATING CHILDREN WITH SEXUALLY ABUSIVE BEHAVIOR PROBLEMS: GUIDELINES FOR CHILD AND PARENT INTERVENTION by Jan Ellen Burton, Lucinda A. Rasmussen, Julie Bradshaw, Barbara J. Christopherson, and Steven C. Huke. (1998). "An extremely readable book that is well-documented and a mine of valuable 'hands on' information. . . . This is a book that all those who work with sexually abusive children or want to work with them must read." *Sharon K. Araji, PhD, Professor of Sociology, University of Alaska, Anchorage*

THE LEARNING ABOUT MYSELF (LAMS) PROGRAM FOR AT-RISK PARENTS: LEARNING FROM THE PAST—CHANGING THE FUTURE by Verna Rickard. (1998). "This program should be a part of the resource materials of every mental health professional trusted with the responsibility of working with 'at-risk' parents." *Terry King, PhD, Clinical Psychologist, Federal Bureau of Prisons, Catlettsburg, Kentucky*

THE LEARNING ABOUT MYSELF (LAMS) PROGRAM FOR AT-RISK PARENTS: HANDBOOK FOR GROUP PARTICIPANTS by Verna Rickard. (1998). "Not only is the LAMS program designed to be educational and build skills for future use, it is also fun!" *Martha Morrison Dore, PhD, Associate Professor of Social Work, Columbia University, New York*

BRIDGING WORLDS: UNDERSTANDING AND FACILITATING ADOLESCENT RECOVERY FROM THE TRAUMA OF ABUSE by Joycee Kennedy and Carol McCarthy. (1998). "An extraordinary survey of the history of child neglect and abuse in America. . . . A wonderful teaching tool at the university level, but should be required reading in high schools as well." *Florabel Kinsler, PhD, BCD, LCSW, Licensed Clinical Social Worker, Los Angeles, California*

CEDAR HOUSE: A MODEL CHILD ABUSE TREATMENT PROGRAM by Bobbi Kendig with Clara Lowry. (1998). "Kendig and Lowry truly . . . realize the saying that we are our brothers' keepers. Their spirit permeates this volume, and that spirit of caring is what always makes the difference for people in painful situations." *Hershel K. Swinger, PhD, Clinical Director, Children's Institute International, Los Angeles, California*

SEXUAL, PHYSICAL, AND EMOTIONAL ABUSE IN OUT-OF-HOME CARE: PREVENTION SKILLS FOR AT-RISK CHILDREN by Toni Cavanagh Johnson and Associates. (1997). "Professionals who make dispositional decisions or who are related to out-of-home care for children could benefit from reading and following the curriculum of this book with children in placements." *Issues in Child Abuse Accusations*

Order a copy of this book with this form or online at:
http://www.haworthpress.com/store/product.asp?sku=5230

DEPRESSION IN NEW MOTHERS
Causes, Consequences, and Treatment Alternatives

_____ in hardbound at $39.95 (ISBN-13: 978-0-7890-1838-0; ISBN-10: 0-7890-1838-1)

_____ in softbound at $24.95 (ISBN-13: 978-0-7890-1839-7; ISBN-10: 0-7890-1839-X)

Or order online and use special offer code HEC25 in the shopping cart.

COST OF BOOKS_____

☐ **BILL ME LATER:** (Bill-me option is good on US/Canada/Mexico orders only; not good to jobbers, wholesalers, or subscription agencies.)
☐ Check here if billing address is different from shipping address and attach purchase order and billing address information.

POSTAGE & HANDLING_____
(US: $4.00 for first book & $1.50 for each additional book)
(Outside US: $5.00 for first book & $2.00 for each additional book)

Signature_____

SUBTOTAL_____

☐ **PAYMENT ENCLOSED:** $_____

IN CANADA: ADD 7% GST_____

☐ **PLEASE CHARGE TO MY CREDIT CARD.**

STATE TAX_____
(NJ, NY, OH, MN, CA, IL, IN, PA, & SD residents, add appropriate local sales tax)

☐ Visa ☐ MasterCard ☐ AmEx ☐ Discover
☐ Diner's Club ☐ Eurocard ☐ JCB

Account # _____

FINAL TOTAL_____
(If paying in Canadian funds, convert using the current exchange rate, UNESCO coupons welcome)

Exp. Date_____

Signature_____

Prices in US dollars and subject to change without notice.

NAME_____

INSTITUTION_____

ADDRESS_____

CITY_____

STATE/ZIP_____

COUNTRY_____ COUNTY (NY residents only)_____

TEL_____ FAX_____

E-MAIL_____

May we use your e-mail address for confirmations and other types of information? ☐ Yes ☐ No
We appreciate receiving your e-mail address and fax number. Haworth would like to e-mail or fax special discount offers to you, as a preferred customer. **We will never share, rent, or exchange your e-mail address or fax number.** We regard such actions as an invasion of your privacy.

Order From Your Local Bookstore or Directly From
The Haworth Press, Inc.
10 Alice Street, Binghamton, New York 13904-1580 • USA
TELEPHONE: 1-800-HAWORTH (1-800-429-6784) / Outside US/Canada: (607) 722-5857
FAX: 1-800-895-0582 / Outside US/Canada: (607) 771-0012
E-mailto: orders@haworthpress.com

For orders outside US and Canada, you may wish to order through your local
sales representative, distributor, or bookseller.
For information, see http://haworthpress.com/distributors

(Discounts are available for individual orders in US and Canada only, not booksellers/distributors.)
PLEASE PHOTOCOPY THIS FORM FOR YOUR PERSONAL USE.
http://www.HaworthPress.com   BOF04